D0678953

the
sex
instruction
manual

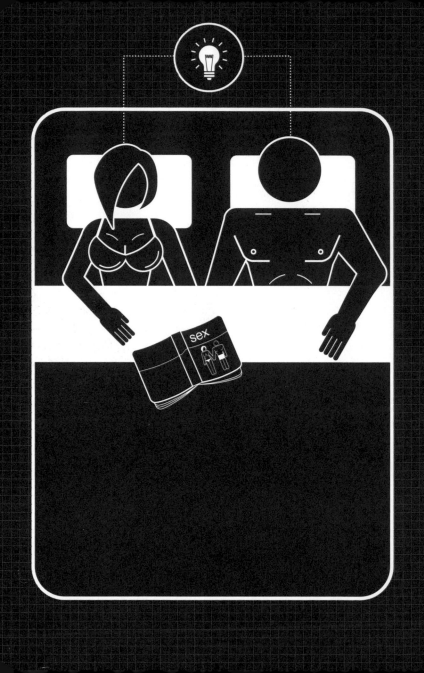

the

sex

instruction manual

ESSENTIAL INFORMATION AND TECHNIQUES
FOR OPTIMUM PERFORMANCE

by Felicia Zopol

Illustrated by Paul Kepple and Scotty Reifsnyder

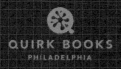

QUIRK BOOKS
PHILADELPHIA

Copyright © 2009 by Quirk Productions, Inc.
Illustrations copyright © 2009 by Headcase Design

All rights reserved. No part of this book may be reproduced in any form without written permission from the publisher.

Library of Congress Cataloging in Publication Number: 2008943529

ISBN: 978-1-59474-336-8
Printed in Canada
Typeset in Swiss

Designed and illustrated by Paul Kepple and Scotty Reifsnyder @ Headcase Design
www.headcasedesign.com
Production management by John J. McGurk

Distributed in North America by Chronicle Books
680 Second Street
San Francisco, CA 94107

10 9 8 7 6 5 4 3 2 1

Quirk Books
215 Church Street
Philadelphia, PA 19106
www.quirkbooks.com

Contents

INTRODUCTION 8

Parts List 11

- The Head 11
- The Body 14

CHAPTER 1: INSTALLATION AND PREPARATION 16

Preparing Your Home 18

- Couch or Loveseat 18
- Other Necessary Components 19

Consumable Seduction Aids 22

Preparing Your Body for Optimum Performance 25

- Warm Up 25
- Sanitizing the Body 28
- Clothes: Your Body's Exterior Sheathing 29
- Other Accessories 32

CHAPTER 2: INITIALIZATION AND FOREPLAY 34

Initialization 36

- Initial Touching 39

Foreplay 41

- Oral Interface (aka Kissing) 41
- Advanced Touching 44
- Breast Stimulation 46
- Alternative Foreplay Activities 50
- Rebooting Strategies 53

CHAPTER 3: MANUAL AND ORAL GENITAL OPERATION 54

Male Genitals 56

- Diagram and Parts List 56

Female Genitals 63

- Diagram and Parts List 63

- Internal Affairs 66
Lubrication 68
Manual Male Genitalia Manipulation 71
- Achieving Full Genital Activation 74
- Shutdown Mode 77
Manual Female Genitalia Manipulation 79
- Achieving Full Genital Activation 82
- Shutdown Mode 83
Oral Genital Operation 85
- Oral Interface with the Male Genitals 86
- Oral Interface with the Female Genitals 92

CHAPTER 4: INTERCOURSE 98
Configuring Your Work Station 100
- The Bed 100
- Other Essential Items 102
- Preparing Your Work Station 107
Protective Devices 109
- Condoms 109
- Female Condoms 116
- Other Intercourse Protection Devices 119
- Longer-Lasting and Permanent Protections 120
Basic Intercourse Mechanics 121
- Core Intercourse Positions 124
- Missionary Variations 125
- Advanced Missionary Variations 128
- Female on Top Variations 130
- Advanced Female on Top Variations 132
- Standing Variations 133
- Advanced Standing Variations 135
- Canine Variations 136
- Advanced Canine Variations 138

- Side-By-Side Variations 139
Anal Intercourse 141
- Hygiene 141
- Anal Foreplay 142
- Penetration 142
- Positions 144
Orgasm 144
- Male Orgasm 145
- Female Orgasm 147
- Enhancing Orgasms 149

CHAPTER 5: ADVANCED SEXUAL INTERFACE 152
Common Alternatives 154
- Unique Alternatives 162
- Determining What Turns You On 163
- Getting Your Partner on Board 166
How to Find a Third Party for a Ménage à Trois 169
How to Develop Your Own Alternative Sexual Activity 172
Troubleshooting 173

CHAPTER 6: SEXUAL ACCESSORIES 176
How to Choose a Vibrator 178
Other Sexual Accessories 181
Caring for Your Accessories 186

CHAPTER 7: MAINTENANCE AND TROUBLESHOOTING 188
Hardware Maintenance 190
- Additional Maintenance 192
- Addressing Sexual Malfunctions 195

APPENDIX 200
INDEX 203
ABOUT THE AUTHOR AND ILLUSTRATORS 208

"It looks like you're

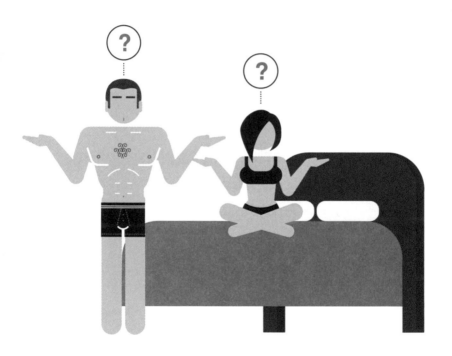

about to have sex.
Would you like help?"

Remember that interactive animated paper clip that used to pop up on your word processing program to help you write a letter? Did you ever wish that something like that could guide you through the often confusing, sometimes cumbersome process of sexual coupling? Maybe not a talking paper clip exactly, but some trusted resource, some, oh, say, authoritative manual that would provide you with the solid, step-by-step instructions you need to make the most out of your sexual activity? The book you are reading now is just such a manual.

Sex is one of the most exciting, pleasurable, and rewarding activities available to the human race—but good luck finding reliable information about it. For most people, the subject is still taboo, and so we stumble through our sexual education via trial, error, and the occasional misleading Web site. Bogus herbal remedies promise to cure every manner of sexual dysfunction, and mass-market pornography—with its cavalcade of freakishly endowed grotesques—does more to distort people's perceptions of what is possible and desirable between lovers than a thousand funhouse mirrors. *The Sex Instruction Manual* is an antidote to all of the rumors and hearsay perpetrated by our consumer culture. It's a guide to maximizing one's pleasure through the proper care, maintenance, and deployment of sexual parts, tools, and techniques.

For convenience and ease of use, this book has been divided into seven sections:

INSTALLATION AND PREPARATION (pages 16–33) offers advice on finding a suitable partner and preparing your home and bedroom.

INITIALIZATION AND FOREPLAY (pages 34–53) offers tips for gently coaxing your partner into the bedroom and guides you through the all-important early stages of lovemaking.

MANUAL AND ORAL GENITAL OPERATION (pages 54–97) presents a series of activities designed to stimulate your partner's most sensitive body parts using nothing more than your ten fingers plus your lips, teeth, and tongue.

INTERCOURSE (pages 98–151) explores the manifold varieties of male–female sexual intercourse, with illustrations of dozens of postures and positions.

ADVANCED SEXUAL INTERFACE (pages 152–175) takes a tour of the outer fringes of sexual interface. It offers a brief introduction to the many kinks and fetishes popular today.

SEXUAL ACCESSORIES (pages 176–187) introduces some of the many devices that people use to increase the pleasure of, and add variety to, their sexual encounters.

MAINTENANCE AND TROUBLESHOOTING (pages 188–199) educates on the many hardware and software glitches that can crash your sex life.

When performed properly, sexual intercourse can provide a lifetime of joy and intimacy. But mastering it takes years of practice and patience. It's not uncommon to experience despair, humiliation, loneliness, and pain in your pursuit of sexual satisfaction. But these feelings are normal and will fade as you become more adept. One day in the not-so-distant future, sexual ecstasy may seem as simple to you as changing a light bulb, turning on the TV, or writing a letter on your computer. Then you will know you have mastered sex.

Now, let's unpack the box, dump the Styrofoam peanuts, and get you started on the road to enjoying your new sex life.

Parts List

Congratulations! Unless you've been the victim of an unfortunate thresher accident, your body is preinstalled with everything you need to achieve total sexual pleasure and fulfillment. Let's review the body parts that you must put into good working order before beginning operation of your sex life. If you or your partner is missing one or more of the parts described, contact a service provider immediately.

The Head

Head: The head is the center of sensory activity and the storage area for a person's unique sexual preferences and behavior. The head may also contain neuroses that can undermine sexual interface and attraction.

Hair: Not present on every model. Tint and thickness may vary. Since hair may be pulled during sexual activity, those wearing toupees may wish to make sure their hairpieces are securely mounted before commencing interface.

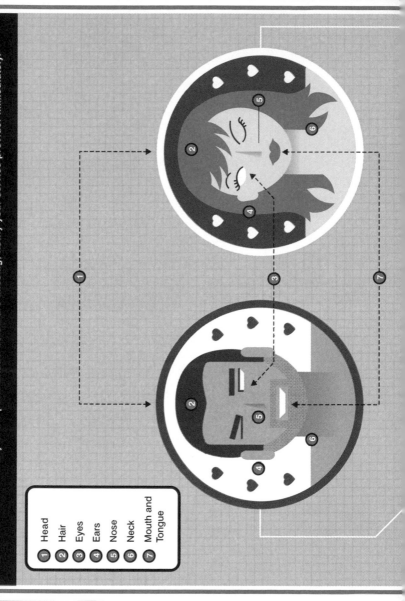

PARTS LIST: If any of the parts shown below are missing, notify your service provider immediately.

1. Head
2. Hair
3. Eyes
4. Ears
5. Nose
6. Neck
7. Mouth and Tongue

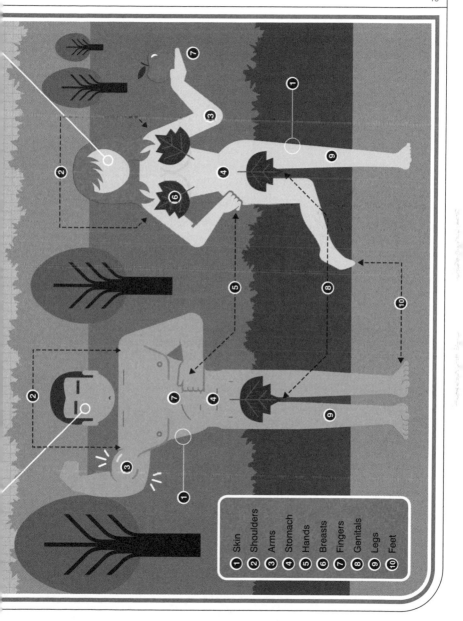

1. Skin
2. Shoulders
3. Arms
4. Stomach
5. Hands
6. Breasts
7. Fingers
8. Genitals
9. Legs
10. Feet

Eyes: Available in brown, gray, green, blue, and other related hues. Watch for slight alterations to indicate level of sexual interest and enjoyment. If eyes glaze over at any point, check for vital signs and begin immediate resuscitation.

Ears: Critical and often underutilized, the ears rarely receive physical attention. However, they can be crucial in alerting you to changes in your partner's physical and psychological state.

Nose: A key sentinel for aromatic signs of sexual attraction and desire.

Mouth and Tongue: Perhaps the most critical sexual hardware component outside the genitals, the mouth plays a significant role in the seduction process and can be used throughout lovemaking in a variety of different ways.

Neck: A highly charged but often overlooked erogenous zone.

The Body

Skin: Covers almost the entire body and acts as a receptor of all physical pleasure.

Shoulders: As the arch of posture, they provide nonverbal clues about a person's sexual confidence and physical state.

Breasts: The most sensitive sexual hardware outside the genitals and two key components of sexual attraction.

Stomach: Holds the body in line during often rigorous sexual activities.

Arms: Critical for hugging and maintaining positioning during intercourse.

Hands: Vital during all stages of intercourse.

Fingers: Along with the tongue, the most skillful and versatile dispensers of pleasure.

Genitals: The epicenter of sexual activity, pleasure, and intimacy.

Legs: An important component in attraction for many people and critical in most intercourse postures.

Feet: A sensitive erogenous zone and the focal point of certain fetishes (see page 155).

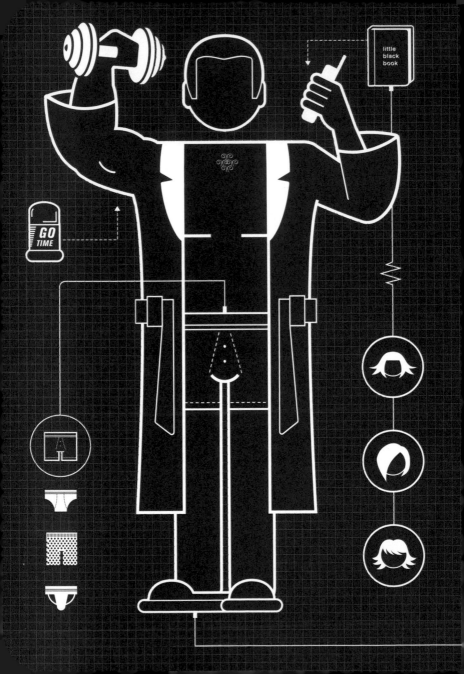

little
black
book

GO
TIME

Chapter 1

Installation and Preparation

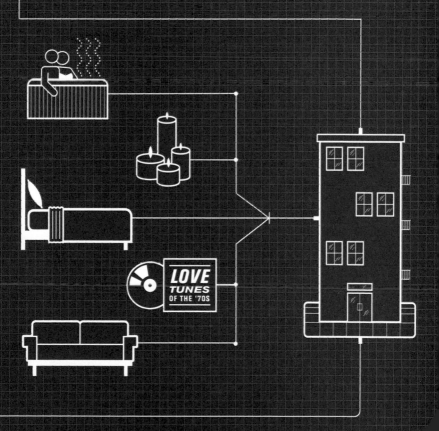

LOVE
TUNES
OF THE '70S

Preparing Your Home

Before attempting sexual interface, make sure your home contains a special area suited for this unique activity. This area will serve as a staging ground for the crucial transitional process between initialization (also known as "seduction"), foreplay, and full sexual interface. Each feature in this location should contribute to the desired mood and atmosphere.

Couch or Loveseat

Evaluate your seating to make sure it is appropriately sized, properly placed, and comfortable.

Size: The couch should be large enough to accommodate two people, but not so large that they can occupy it while sitting more than an arm's length apart.

Placement: Situate the couch in an easily accessible area that lies outside the room's major pathways (e.g., door-to-bedroom, door-to-kitchen, kitchen-to-bathroom). If you have roommates, the couch should be placed in a more remote area of the room where you can continue initialization without being interrupted by a roommate's unexpected arrival.

Comfort: The couch should be comfortable and relaxing. Test the cushions to ensure they are not so soft that you and your partner sink into them, thus limiting mobility. Excessive sinkage can undermine easy maneuvering and fluent repositioning during seduction and foreplay.

Other Necessary Components

Beverage Preparation Center: An alcoholic beverage helps relax many people and allows them to be more receptive to the seduction process, lessening their stress and lowering their inhibitions. Stock a table or cabinet with several varieties of liquor (vodka, whiskey, gin, scotch, rum), plus beer and wine. Include "mixers," such as sodas and juices for the liquor. The mixers can also serve as alternative beverages for those who do not consume alcohol.

Table: Place a low, sturdy table in front or to the side of the couch to place drinks and other items upon.

Recorded-Music Playing Device: Musical vibrations can help set the mood and relax a person while covering distracting sounds emanating from outside or surrounding domiciles. Include a wide variety of recorded music to cover an array of music tastes.

Lighting Apparatus: Remove lamps or light bulbs that cast light that is too bright or direct. This type of light can cause a person to seize up or become overly self-conscious. Replace high-watt bulbs with low-wattage models and rearrange lamps to cast soft, indirect light, which creates a more relaxing atmosphere.

EXPERT TIP: *Equip your seduction location with an enjoyable alternate activity, such as a game or a television. Many people are prone to seizing up when seduction efforts become too direct. Engaging in the alternative activity for a while after arrival will help relieve tension so that both parties are more open to sexual interface.*

COUCH ESSENTIALS

1. Size
2. Placement
3. Comfort

OTHER HOME PREPARATION ELEMENTS TO CONSIDER

4. Recorded-music playing device
5. Beverage preparation center
6. Lighting apparatus
7. Table

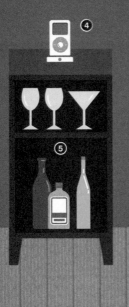
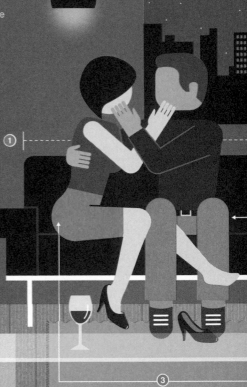

HOME PREPARATION: Be sure to establish a staging area for seduction

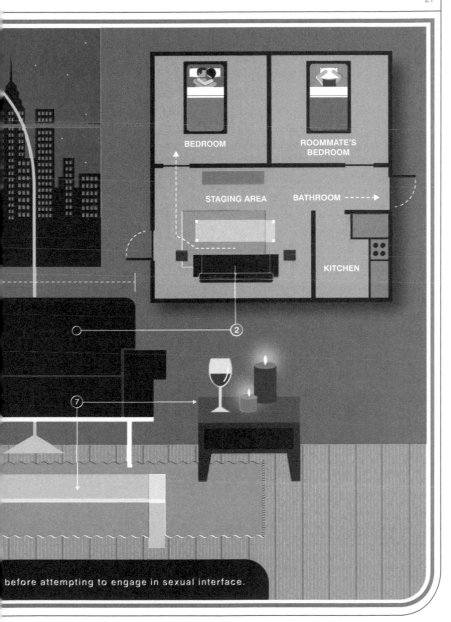

BEDROOM

ROOMMATE'S
BEDROOM

STAGING AREA

BATHROOM - - - - →

KITCHEN

②

⑦

before attempting to engage in sexual interface.

Consumable Seduction Aids

Known in common parlance as aphrodisiacs, certain foodstuffs have acquired a reputation as sex enhancers. Although the veracity of such claims can almost never be proved scientifically, you may feel that the mere proffering of these consumables serves as an aid to seduction.

■ *Oysters* have long had a reputation as being aphrodisiacs. According to legend, Casanova ate dozens of them every morning. Although most researchers have dismissed the effects as purely psychological, these effects should not be underestimated. Simply put: Many people say oysters remind them of genitals.

■ *Coconut* has acquired a reputation as a sex enhancer, especially in the Caribbean. Research indicates that coconut is loaded with compounds that boost the action of testosterone.

■ *Truffles*, the highly prized edible fungi, produce androstenol, a musky pheromone found in the saliva of boars. That explains why pigs are turned on by them—but what about humans? It may have something to do with the chi-chi cachet associated with the truffle's high price and legendarily difficult extraction.

■ *Durian* is a popular Southeast Asian tree fruit; it is considered an aphrodisiac in Indonesia, where aficionados boast that "when the durian fruit comes down, the skirts come up!" You may want to offer this treat in small doses, however, since durian literally smells and tastes like rotting garbage.

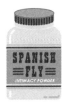

■ *Spanish Fly* is a bitter, vile-tasting powder made from the ground bodies of dead beetles. If that alone doesn't make you reconsider sharing some with your date, be aware that it induces priapism (enormous, painful erections that won't go away) and can cause permanent kidney damage and even death. Nevertheless, for centuries it was slipped into drinks as the ultimate pre-orgy icebreaker. Today, Spanish fly is illegal almost everywhere, so whatever you're buying is most likely just cayenne powder in a capsule.

Other Foods Reputed to Have Aphrodisiac Effects:

■ Arugula	■ Kelp	■ Mussels	■ Artichokes
■ Chocolate	■ Onions	■ Turtle Eggs	

NICE PACKAGE: Appealing physical appearances are vital to sexual interface.

STEREOTYPICALLY UNATTRACTIVE PACKAGE

MALE

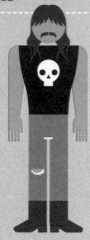

FEMALE

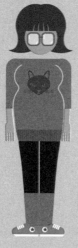

STEREOTYPICALLY ATTRACTIVE PACKAGE

MALE

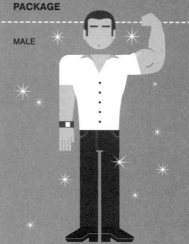

FEMALE

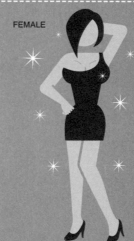

*NOTE:
Images are based on stereotypes. Everyone has his or her own personal taste.

Preparing Your Body for Optimum Performance

Your body is of primary importance when it comes to sexual interface. Taking good care of yourself and presenting yourself as a desirable and attractive package will ease seduction efforts with your partner.

Warm Up

Opportunities for sexual interface can arise when you least expect them. In most cases, you won't be able to complete these stretches and exercises immediately beforehand, so perform them regularly at home. They will help keep you flexible and ready to achieve optimum performance in the bedroom.

Neck: Bend your chin toward your chest and hold for 30 seconds. Bend your head back as far as it will go, with your chin pointing toward the ceiling, and hold for 30 seconds. Tilt your right ear toward your right shoulder, then left, holding each stretch for 30 seconds. Repeat series 5 times.

Groin: Sit on the floor, placing the bottoms of your feet together in front and your knees pointing out to either side. Rest your elbows against your knees and slowly push them toward the floor as far as they will go. Hold stretch for 20 seconds and repeat 5 times. Extend both legs in a V shape in front of you. Slowly and simultaneously move both legs as far out to the sides as they will extend without discomfort. Hold for 20 seconds and repeat 3 times. Bend your upper body toward the floor as far as it will extend and hold for 15 seconds. Repeat 5 times.

Cardio: Before stretching your muscles, warm them up by some light jogging or fastwalking. This will also get your heart muscle working and warmed up. Dancing is also an excellent warm-up activity, for it employs many of the same motions and muscles used in foreplay and sexual interface.

Lower back: Lie on the floor and bend your legs so the bottoms of your feet touch. Stretch your knees to either side and as far down as you can without discomfort. Hold for 30 seconds and repeat 5 times.

Legs: Sit on the floor and extend your legs straight in front of you, then bend forward from the waist as far as you can. Hold for 10 seconds; repeat 5 times. Raise your upper body off the floor, keeping your legs stretched out in front of you. Loop a towel around the back of your upper right foot. Holding one end of the towel in each hand, pull your foot as far as you can and hold for 30 seconds. Repeat 5 times with each leg. Lie on your stomach, with your upper body raised slightly off the floor and supported on your elbows. Bend your knee and bring your right foot as close to your buttocks as you can. Hold for 30 seconds. Switch to the left leg. Repeat 5 times with each leg.

Feet: The foot muscles are the secret workhorses of many sexual activities. Unprepared feet often cramp before, during, and after sexual interface. Start by rubbing the long muscle on your instep, between the heel and arch. Move each toe gently back and forth and up and down, as far as is comfortable. Firmly grip the rail of a staircase and stand on the lower step, with the back half of your feet hanging over the edge. Shift your weight to your heels, stretching your soles and the back of your legs.

Upper back: Stand and extend both arms over your head as high as you can. Hold for 30 seconds; release. Repeat 5 times. Join your hands over your head, interlocking fingers, and turn your palms upward. Stretch your arms as high as you can. Hold for 30 seconds. Repeat 5 times.

Pelvis: Standing with your hands on your hips and knees slightly bent, move your pelvis forward and back 25 times, quickening the motion as you proceed. In the same position, roll your hips from side to side, then in a figure eight 25 times in each direction.

Bend over: Bend at the waist as far as you can, with your fingers extending toward the floor. Hold for 10 seconds, then rise back up and repeat 15 times.

Mouth and jaw: This stretch will help you avoid embarrassing and inconvenient jaw cramps during sexual activities. Slowly open your mouth as wide as possible, as if to yawn. Hold the stretch for 10 seconds. Repeat 5 times.

Tongue: Slowly stick out your tongue as far as you can. Keeping it extended, roll it around the edge of your lips 10 times, then reverse direction for 10 more revolutions. With tongue extended, flick the tip up and down, then back and forth 10 times.

Sanitizing the Body

It is important to sanitize the body before attempting any kind of sexual interface. Failure to do so could cause your partner to enter shutdown mode.

[1] *Bathe or shower.* Submerge yourself in clean water in a bath or shower. Sanitize your entire surface area using a pleasant-smelling soap or body wash. Make sure to disinfect and deodorize your armpits, crotch, feet, buttocks, and other areas that produce strong odors.

[2] If applicable, *wash all the hair on your cranium.* Apply products, such as conditioners, that make your hair more appealing and easy to manipulate. Use combs, a brush, and your hands to reshape your hair into a formation that accentuates or hides your facial features in an advantageous manner.

[3] *Sanitize the mouth.* Thoroughly scrub your oral area, clearing it of all food particles and residues with a toothbrush and toothpaste. Rinse your mouth with a pleasant-smelling mouthwash or breath mint.

[4] *Reodorize.* Add aromatic flourishes such as perfumes and colognes designed to please your partner.

⚠ *WARNING: Do not overload any part of your body with an aromatic enhancer. A high concentration of perfume or cologne can actually overwhelm and cause your partner to enter shut-down mode.*

Clothes: Your Body's Exterior Sheathing

Though full sexual interface usually involves the removal of all or most of your clothing, your ability to convince your partner to enter into sexual interface will largely depend on how effectively you package your body. As a general guideline, wear clothing that clearly communicates your particular "brand" and is likely to attract the type of person you are looking to seduce.

[1] *Underwear.* Apply a first layer of clothing to cover your sexual hardware. Chose appropriate underwear as well as bras and lingerie that are especially flattering and enticing. Be sure to select items that also keep your hardware from overheating or getting chilled, depending on the weather.

⚠ *WARNING: Eschew codpieces, merkins, and other prefabricated articles designed to artificially enhance or conceal sexual hardware. Truth in advertising is always the best policy.*

[2] *Shape.* Dress yourself in a layer of stylish, age-appropriate clothing that highlights your best features and downplays your trouble spots. Pay special attention to sexually enticing areas such as the buttocks, chest, and legs.

[3] *Texture.* Wear soft, luxurious, and natural fabrics such as cashmere, silk, and pima cotton, which may make a partner want to get closer to you.

[4] *Color.* Select colors that flatter your skin tone, eyes, and hair color. If you're not sure which tones suit you best, test different ones on several occasions. Note the responses of other people and refine your seduction wardrobe accordingly.

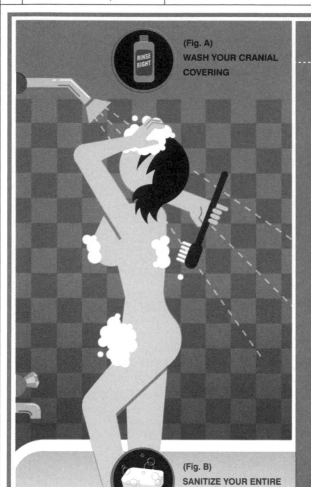

(Fig. A)
WASH YOUR CRANIAL COVERING

RINSE RIGHT

(Fig. B)
SANITIZE YOUR ENTIRE SURFACE USING SOAP

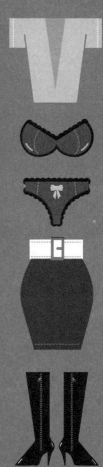

HER SHEATHING

SANITIZING AND SHEATHING: Maintaining your outward appearance

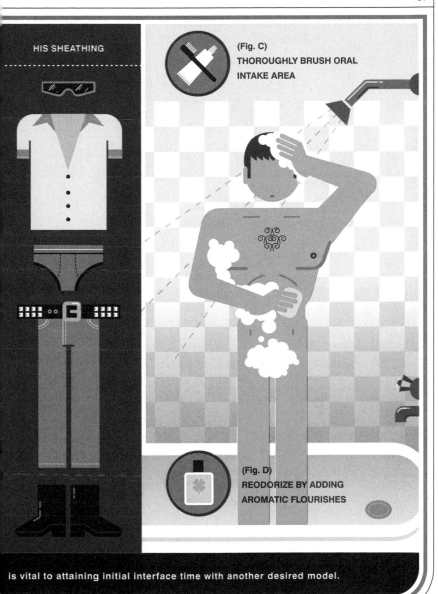

HIS SHEATHING

(Fig. C)
THOROUGHLY BRUSH ORAL
INTAKE AREA

(Fig. D)
REODORIZE BY ADDING
AROMATIC FLOURISHES

is vital to attaining initial interface time with another desired model.

[5] *Shoes.* Some people have highly developed sartorial sensors that disqualify prospects equipped with substandard footwear. Always wear your best available and most appropriate shoes.

[6] *Skin.* Temperature permitting, wear clothing that exposes portions of your skin in sexually significant body areas such as the neck, legs, arms, and midriff.

EXPERT TIP: Including extra nonessential items in your look can help alert your partner that you are style confident and desirable. Such items can help jump-start seduction by providing a casual conversation opener.

Other Accessories

Neckwear. A flattering necktie, scarf, kerchief, or necklace draws attention to the sexually charged bodily transition zone between your head and torso. Men may wish to steer clear of ascots, dickies, or other articles of clothing that have acquired a foppish or anachronistic cachet.

Timepiece. A stylish, expensive watch displays your advanced sense of fashion and economic stature. It can also provide an interested prospect with an excuse to ask you for the correct time—a longstanding conversation/pick-up jump-starter.

Bracelets and rings. These items can symbolize sexual loyalty to another person, but they also attract interest and enhance the visual presentation of the sexually charged hand area. Note that in rare cases a wedding band or ring can have the seemingly paradoxical effect of encouraging, rather than dissuading, advances from would-be sexual partners. There may be a "forbidden fruit" dynamic at play. Also, an overly ostentatious display of jewelry (or "bling," to use common parlance) can have a down-market connotation in certain circles. Consider toning down (or amping up) your use of such items, depending on the type of partner you wish to attract.

Earrings. Whether sparkly or dangling, these accoutrements can enhance facial features and help draw the attention of potential partners.

Body piercings. These can draw attention to your body but also signal willingness to engage in certain alternative sexual activities (see chapter 5). In almost all instances, genital piercings should be kept concealed at all times while in public.

Headwear. Hats can enhance your facial features or cover up unflattering hair malfunctions. Choose a hat that is stylish and age appropriate and coordinates with the rest of your outfit. Avoid overly cumbersome or obviously unnatural-looking hairpieces, wigs, and hair extensions (if possible). By doing so, you will avoid having to explain or remove them later, when intimacy forces your hand.

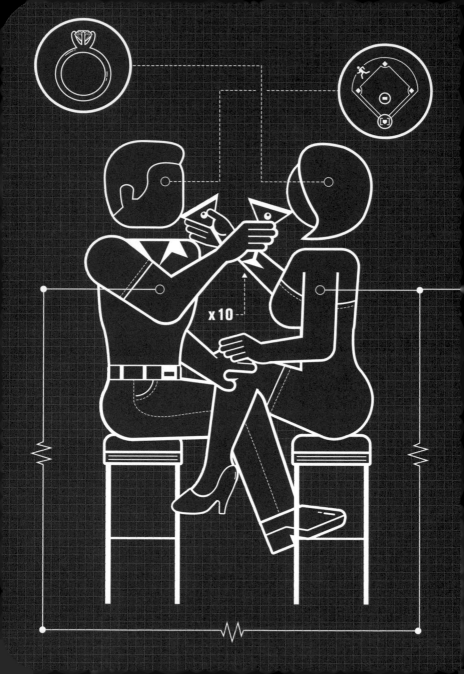

Chapter 2

Intialization and Foreplay

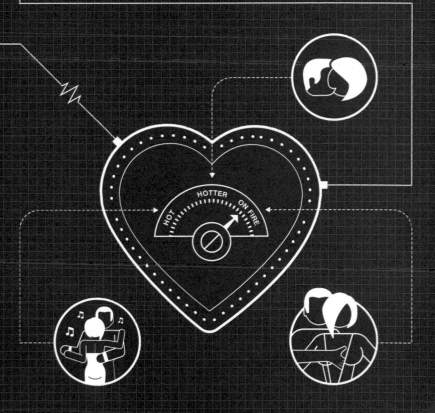

Initialization

Even after mutual sexual attraction has been established, most people still require a process of initialization (also known as "booting up" or "seduction") in which they are drawn slowly and willingly into sexual interface. In general, this is accomplished by various demonstrations of sexual appeal that activate both partners' erotic desires. But exactly what works will vary widely from person to person and usually requires customization to reflect individual tastes. Here are some basic seduction activities and techniques that you can experiment with and customize.

■ *Conversing.* Discuss topics other than sex, which will help the other person relax and get to know you better. Ask about his or her life, day, experiences, and aspirations.

EXPERT TIP: Listening is the key to effective communication. Most people want to feel that you value their opinions. So listen closely and make sure your responses reflect that you understand and appreciate what the person is saying. Listening will help you learn about the person's interests and what is likely to activate him or her. It will also help you learn more reasons for your attraction.

■ *Gazing.* Look directly into the person's eyes while talking. This simple technique can either be incredibly seductive or alert you that the person is not ready for seduction.

■ *Dancing.* Moving your body rhythmically to musical vibrations helps simultaneously relax your partner and activate erotic desire, providing the opportunity to signal sexual interest.

■ *Tabooing.* If the other person is reluctant to continue with sexual interface for moral reasons, try engaging in a mostly innocuous yet still morally questionable activity. Perform a practical joke on a mutual acquaintance. Play hooky from work together. Steal a neighbor's lawn ornament. Indulging in and enjoying such mildly dishonorable pursuits may help your partner loosen up or become excited, opening the door to sexual interface.

⚠ *WARNING: Coaxing is acceptable, but do not exert verbal pressure or complain if the other person is not ready to proceed with foreplay. Effective interface requires trust, comfort, and mutual enthusiasm. Engage in activities that will help the person achieve those states with you instead of undermining them through negativity.*

■ *Massaging.* Extended, intense touching and manipulation of a particular body area is a great way to help a person relax and affirm a more positive relationship between you. Massages require patience and a certain level of knowledge, but you can gain much of that knowledge through experience. Concentrate your efforts on one part of the body. (The neck, shoulders, upper back, and feet are popular locations.) Begin rubbing the area, focusing on the largest muscles. Start gently, then experiment with various motions, areas, and pressure to explore which applications the person enjoys most. Massage can take many years to perfect, but with practice, and by paying attention to feedback, you should be able to administer an effective and much-appreciated massage on your first try. Note: Avoid massaging the genitalia unless specifically prompted to do so.

■ *Head or Scalp Massaging.* Because it houses the erotic software you must activate for effective interface, a person's head is particularly vulnerable to the kind of muscle tension that can frustrate erotic desire. As a consequence, you need to ensure that this area is functioning properly. Rub your partner's forehead, starting your thumbs in its center and pushing them slowly outward. Continue across the temples. Use all your fingers to rub the top of the head, beginning at the front and moving to the rear. Gently stroke the back of the cranial apparatus. Gauge the person's feedback to see which area or areas crave the most attention, and repeat your efforts there.

⚠ **EXPERT TIP:** *A person complaining of a headache is usually sending you a signal of reluctance to enter into or continue with sexual interface. You can test the validity or overcome this objection with the offer of a long, gentle head rub.*

■ *Cuddling.* Sitting or reclining on a couch or mattress and interlocking arms and legs can relax a partner and help form a bond of trust between you. The posture also serves as a good starting point for foreplay activities.

⚠ **EXPERT TIP:** *Letting a person observe you doing something well can be an even more effective seduction technique than direct efforts. Skillfully perform a non-sex-related act in your dwelling or public space. Time-honored competencies that have been showcased in this manner include the aforementioned dancing as well as cooking (bonus points awarded for demonstration of esoteric techniques or mastery of arcane/trendy ethnic cuisines), skating (ice or roller), bowling, drag racing, or skeet shooting.*

Visual Cues That Your Partner Is Ready for Sexual Interface

■ Moving Next to You
■ Opening Posture
■ Staring
■ Outer Clothing Removal

■ Playing with Your Hair
■ Lip Licking
■ Touching
■ Lap Sitting

Initial Touching

Once you and your partner have both activated your mutual desire through seduction and settled into a location suitable for sexual activities, it is usually best to initiate a final transitional step of light, strategic touching. This stimulation of minor erotic sensors will help you and your partner heighten the level of activation, communicate, confirm intentions, build trust, and prepare for stimulation of major sexual sensors through foreplay.

As you engage in initial touching activities, focus on the other person's eyes. Such "eye contact" will not only help you gauge responses to your touching but can also heighten arousal.

Hands: Stroke the back of your partner's hand with your fingertips. Gently grasp one or both hands in your own. Touch your lips to the back of the hand. Stroke and nibble individual fingers.

Arms: Run your fingers down the outside of your partner's arms. Move gently to the arms' sensitive undersides.

Shoulders and Back: Stroke your partner's shoulders and upper back with your hands. Gently squeeze and knead the large muscles located there.

Full Arm Encirclement: Loop your arms around your partner at the top, middle, or lower part of the back until your arms overlap behind. Hold this position.

EXPERT TIP: Encircling your partner from behind, instead of in front, can be highly erotic. This approach can also allow you to move more easily into stimulation of various erogenous zones.

⚠️ **WARNING:** *If the person is too large to encircle fully, extend your arms as far as you can and refrain from commenting on your inability to achieve complete encirclement. But if the person is, for example, a male body builder proud of his thick torso, remarking on your inability to fully enclose him in your arms could bolster his confidence and increase arousal.*

Feet: Place your feet so that they touch the other person's feet. Run your toes up and down the person's lower leg region. Intertwine the lower legs. Note: This maneuver is best performed after removing your shoes, although some males may find the stimulation supplied by, say, a stiletto heel erotically charged. At no time should you execute this maneuver while wearing cleats.

Hair: Move your hand over the person's head and run your fingers through the hair. If your partner responds favorably, run your fingers the full length of the head, starting at the top and moving downward. In the case of bald individuals or those with shaved heads, substitute gentle stroking of the hairless area. Vocal exhortations about how sexy you find a bald head (if genuine) may prove invaluable in assuaging any feelings of follicular inadequacy the other person may feel.

⚠️ **WARNING:** *Confirm, through visual inspection, whether the person is wearing a wig or toupee before proceeding with hair stimulation activities. Vigorous or even moderate contact could lead to hairpiece displacement, and a total sexual shutdown may occur. Also refrain from hair touching if the person has natural hair configured in an especially complex or delicate manner, such as a bouffant or pompadour.*

Foreplay

For the majority of people under the majority of circumstances, the transition from initial activation of arousal to full sexual interface requires a period of warm-up activity known as "foreplay." This process involves stimulation of various erotic sensors in order to prepare for full genital-on-genital activity.

The exact means and amount of time required to accomplish this transition vary from person to person. Some need only a few minutes; others require months of intermittent foreplay prior to full interface. Fortunately, these foreplay activities can be highly rewarding in themselves.

Oral Interface (aka Kissing)

Direct mouth-to-mouth contact marks the first official stage of sexual interface for most people. The mouth contains numerous sensors and plays a role in a wide variety of sexual activities. Adjoining mouths offers pleasurable stimulation and a direct link to subsequent sexual activities.

Shortly before you begin mouth hookup, consume a piece of candy, a breath mint, or a flavored drink. This step is especially important if you smoke or chew tobacco; you definitely wish to avoid evoking the sensation of "licking an ashtray." Offer one to the other person as well. Doing so will help the person warm up the mouth and discreetly eliminate unpleasant breath odors. It will also spare you from later having to embarrass the person with a request to ameliorate unacceptable breath during hookup activities.

Once you are ready for full-on oral interface, follow these steps.

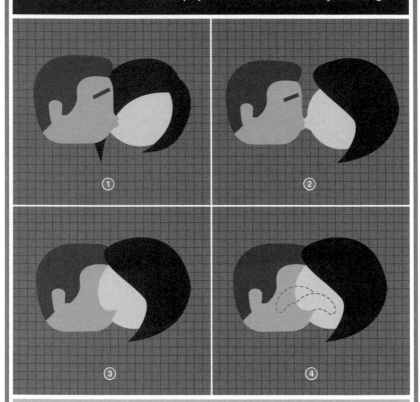

ORAL INTERFACE: Wait for proper authorization before orally interfacing!

(1)

(2)

(3)

(4)

A FEW REMINDERS TO KEEP IN MIND WHEN INTERFACING COMMENCES:

1. Pucker your lips.
2. Gently place mouth on partner's mouth.
3. Press your mouths together and hold.
4. Gently push your tongue into your partner's mouth.

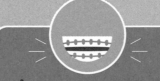

⚠ CAUTION: Be cautious when orally interfacing with partners wearing a dental apparatus.

[1] Pucker your lips and place your mouth on sensitive areas near your partner's mouth, moving from cheeks to forehead to ears. If the person does not pull away or protest, you are probably ready for the next step.

[2] Gently place your mouth on your partner's mouth. Push the fleshier, moister inside of your lips forward so they make contact with the outside, then inside, of his or her lips.

[3] Press your mouths together and hold. Press your lips forward so they make contact with the inside of the other person's lips. Move your lips and mouth slightly up and down and side to side. Alternate the pressure and the parts of the person's lips you come in contact with. Adjust the positioning of your head and neck to find new, more pleasing angles of contact.

⚠ *WARNING: Be more gentle and cautious when orally interfacing with partners wearing a dental apparatus such as braces or dentures. Vigorous interface could cause injury to either party or may result in the dislocation of the apparatus. If both parties are wearing dental apparatus, exert particular caution, for such interface may result in the fusing of the devices, which will likely lead to discomfort, the cessation of interface activities, and an embarrassing trip to the emergency room.*

[4] Gently push your tongue through your lips and into your partner's mouth. Swirl your tongue around the entryway and against the person's tongue. Move it slowly deeper into the person's mouth and across and around his or her tongue.

[**5**] Experiment with different postures and lip and tongue motions until you locate a few that you both find pleasing. Repeat them randomly, moving from one to the other and back again.

⚠ **EXPERT TIP:** *Remember to come up for air every once in a while. No one enjoys kissing when they can't breathe. Also, be sure to use the middle part of the tongue in your kiss because of the large number of sensitive nerve endings there.*

Advanced Touching

The transition from mouth-to-mouth interface to more advanced foreplay activities can be eased by stimulation of various minor erotic sensors. Though it may require some attention and practice, these efforts are usually most effective when performed while maintaining mouth contact.

Midriff: Brush your fingers over the person's stomach. Move them slowly down the sides, from top to bottom. Gently grasp either side of the midriff. They aren't called "love handles" for nothing.

Buttocks: Trace your fingers around the outside of the person's buttocks. Cup each buttock in your palms. Gently squeeze each cheek. Squeeze the cheeks together and move them gently up and down against each other. Avoid tapping out a recognizable rhythm, such as a conga line or Bo Diddley beat, as this may prove distracting.

Back of Knee: Gently move your fingertips across the soft flesh behind the knee. This area is highly sensitive, so do not press hard into the knee joint or linger there too long.

Thighs: Lightly rub the outside and top of the thigh. Move your fingertips to the inside of the thighs for maximum stimulation impact.

Neck: Brush your fingertips on the side of the person's neck and then move your mouth to the area. Kiss and apply pressure on the long muscles on the sides of the neck.

⚠ **WARNING:** *Avoid applying pressure with your hands or mouth to the bulge at the front middle of the person's neck. This "Adam's apple" is highly sensitive, and pressing against it can cause the person great discomfort and may even interrupt breathing, an essential function for continuation of sexual interface. Blocking airflow in order to heighten sexual arousal, also known as autoerotic asphyxiation, or "gasping," is strongly discouraged—and certainly not a wise move at this stage of foreplay. It may serve to frighten and/or kill your partner. Also note that prolonged application of pressure to and sucking on other parts of the neck can lead to bruising or the rupture of small blood vessels beneath the skin, causing a dark spot, or "hickey," to appear on the person's neck and remain for several days.*

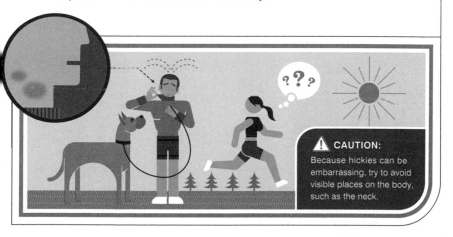

⚠ **CAUTION:**
Because hickies can be embarrassing, try to avoid visible places on the body, such as the neck.

Breast Stimulation

One of the most sensitive and erotically charged pieces of hardware on the human body, breasts play an important role in sexual activities. Though female mammaries get most of the attention, men's breasts are also highly sensitive and can aid greatly in activating sexual arousal.

[1] Trace your fingers around the outside of the breast while the female is still wearing clothing.

[2] Cup one breast in your hand. Gently squeeze.

[3] Reach underneath the person's upper-body clothing to touch the breast area directly. If the female is wearing a secondary layer of clothing, such as a brassiere, rub around the breast area for a moment through the brassiere, then remove it.

⚠ *WARNING: Brassieres can be deceptively difficult to remove. Delays in their removal can lead to frustration, embarrassment, and sexual system failure. Bras are held together by hooks located at either the front centers between the cups or in the middle of the back straps. This hook can be disengaged by pushing the two sides of the bra material around it toward each other and slightly twisting one side until the hook is loosened and then dislodged. Though simple, the exact motion of the maneuver may vary slightly among types. Instead of trying to casually remove the brassiere with one hand, it is usually best to use both hands, pausing momentarily in your other foreplay efforts to concentrate on the maneuver.*

[4] Once you have disengaged the breasts from their packaging, repeat the cupping and tracing maneuvers you performed earlier.

BREAST UNITS: Sensitive and erotically charged pieces of hardware

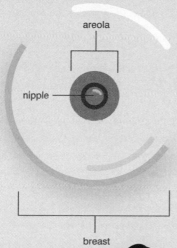

areola

nipple

breast

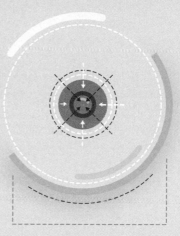

Breast units are usually housed in a bra, which may be difficult to remove.

TECHNIQUES FOR BREAST STIMULATION:

 Apply fingertip action

 Apply gentle cupping or squeezing action

 Apply licking or tongue flicking action

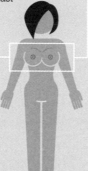

NOTE:
Men's breasts are also sensitive and can be a source of pleasure for him.

WARNING DO NOT:

 Fiddle or tune

 Bite or chomp

 Grab or latch

[**5**] If your hair is long enough, let it fall over the female's breasts. Move your head back and forth so that your hair brushes across the nipples and other parts of the breast.

[**6**] With the lightest possible touch, trace a fingertip around the outside of the nipples. Find a motion that pleases the female and repeat a few times.

EXPERT TIP: Lubricate your fingers before applying them to the nipple. Moisture eases movement and intensifies sensation. Because you may also be applying your mouth to the area, use an edible lubricant. Or simply stick your finger in your mouth or the female's mouth to moisten them with saliva.

[**7**] Place all your fingertips around the outside of the nipple and then slowly move them inward while raising them slightly, as if you are gently lifting the nipple.

[**8**] Move your mouth onto the breast. Extend your tongue to trace and flick it around the dark area around the nipple, or areola. Use your fingers on the other breast as you do this.

WARNING: During stimulation procedures, most nipples will become engorged with blood, making them harder and two to three times larger. Do not become alarmed. This response is normal and signals approval, not injury, malfunction, or imminent bursting.

[**9**] Once the nipple is erect, move your tongue up and down, starting from the base of the nipple and moving to its tip. Flick the tip of your tongue over the tip of the nipple. Trace circles around it, reversing direction after every few revolutions.

⚠ **WARNING:** *Because they are so sensitive, most breasts cannot endure constant attention in one area, particularly the nipple. Vary your stimulation efforts and locations around the breast and nipples to avoid overstimulation and interruption of arousal. Excessive fixation on this body part by males, often accompanied by "baby talk" or plaintive requests for milk, can quickly become creepy and off-putting for females who do not share this nursing fantasy.*

[**10**] Stimulate the underside of the breast with your tongue. This erotically charged area is often overlooked. Avoid the area, however, if you suspect that your partner may be equipped with synthetic breast enhancers; breast-enhancement surgery will have resulted in a scar, and its discovery will likely cause discomfort and embarrassment for your partner.

⚠ **WARNING:** *A significant percentage of females come equipped with breast-enhancement devices that make their breasts rounder and more prominent. You can identify these synthetic breasts by noting their odd texture, preternatural firmness, and lack of sag or jiggling, even when the female is lying down or moving quickly. Refrain from commenting on the synthetic nature of these specimens or the surgery scars. The female obviously went to great expense and discomfort to acquire the enhancers, so limit remarks about them, perhaps simply noting how impressed you are by their beauty, girth, and appearance. Also note that these devices tend to make a female's breasts less sensitive and may require more vigorous and prolonged activation efforts.*

[**11**] If possible, push the breasts together so you can attend to both nipples at once within your mouth or by flicking your tongue from side to side.

What the Breasts Are Not

■ The breasts are not radio dials. Avoid excessive "fiddling" or "tuning" of the nipples, as this action can cause irritation.

■ The breasts are not your dinner. Gentle suction and light nibbling on the nipples is fine. Hard biting and indiscriminate chomping is not.

■ The breasts are not your lifeline. Do not grab or latch onto your partner's breasts, even in the throes of passion, unless specifically directed to do so. If you are male, treat them with the same courtesy and respect with which you would want your two testicles to be treated.

■ The breasts are not the same for everyone. This is especially important to keep in mind when your partner is a female with very sensitive breasts, which can be caused by pregnancy, menstrual cycle, or other biological factors. Making eye contact, listening for responses, and asking your partner what she prefers are the most effective ways of determining whether your breastwork is proving arousing, or is merely nettlesome.

Alternative Foreplay Activities

Sometimes an indirect or unexpected approach can prove more effective in fully activating sexual arousal. Try these activities to stimulate your partner in surprising ways.

Feathering: Take a long, soft feather and trace it over the person's sensitive areas such as the lips, cheeks, legs, stomach, breasts, neck, etc. Try a feather in each hand working on separate parts of the person's body.

Featherdusting: A cleaning apparatus equipped with dozens of feathers multiplies the titillations provided by a single feather. Avoid used featherdusters, which will spread more dirt than pleasurable stimulation.

Silking: Rub a piece of silk or other smooth, soft fabric across sensitive parts of the body.

Gaming: Play strip poker. Or try one of the numerous sexually themed board games available. Or just eroticize a regular game such as tag or Yahtzee. The resulting fun and competition can reduce inhibition and activate arousal.

⚠ *EXPERT TIP: The old childhood game of tickling can prove highly effective in activating a sluggish partner or relaxing a tense one. During initial touching activities, note any areas, such as the abdomen or soles of the feet, that when touched cause the person to recoil and giggle. If necessary, return to these areas for vigorous tickling efforts with your fingertips or a feather.*

Stretching: Take turns helping each other stretch out legs, arms, and backs. These activities will lead to sensual touching as well as deeper, more satisfying stretching that will help activate arousal and prepare for sex.

Co-Eating: Feed each other a spoonful of cake. Lick whipped cream off each other's chests. Pour liquid refreshment on each other's midriffs, then lap it up. These and other shared eating activities stimulate the lips and tongue as well as other portions of the body.

⚠ *WARNING: You may be considering a trip to the local sex shop to purchase edible underwear, an undergarment made of gelatin and artificial flavoring that can be consumed during foreplay. Bear in mind that edible undergarments made with sugar should be kept clear of the female genitalia, as they may increase the risk of yeast infection. Also, remember that the term* edible *is being used very loosely here; eating this underwear is akin to consuming a hundred-year-old fruit roll-up.*

Relocating: Moving to a different setting can help relax and/or excite. If the person seems tense in the current situation, try moving to a more comfortable place, one that is private and/or familiar to your partner. If the person seems bored and disengaged, try an altogether unexpected setting, such as a kitchen countertop, a forest, an alley, or a stairwell. Such surprises may serve to heighten arousal.

Blindfolding: Covering a person's eyes with a bandana or cloth, then manually stimulating various hardware units, can enhance the sensation of touch and anticipation. This exercise also builds excitement and trust.

Stripteasing: Slowly and sensually undressing yourself and each other helps heighten anticipation and hardware awareness. It also provides numerous opportunities for stimulation with pieces of clothing (e.g., slowly pulling a stocking up and down a person's leg).

Bathing: Climbing into a bath, shower, or hot tub together will not only afford you the chance to undress each other but also provide myriad arousal

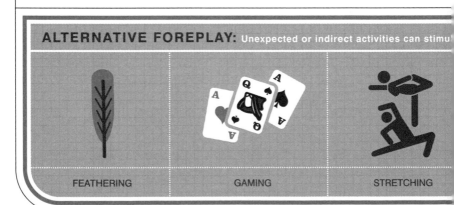

ALTERNATIVE FOREPLAY: Unexpected or indirect activities can stimu

FEATHERING GAMING STRETCHING

opportunities. Warm water relaxes the body and the mind, helping deactivate blocks to erotic enjoyment. A shower stream can be aimed onto the breasts, lips, buttocks, or other erotically charged areas. Being completely naked together also opens up the full range of foreplay activities and helps ease tensions and insecurities.

Rebooting Strategies

Foreplay activities do not always have the intended effect. During their application the other person may lose, rather than gain, interest in further interface. This loss of interest may be due to ineffective technique, distraction, anxiety, or the belief that you have moved too quickly from seduction to full interface. Whatever the cause, if you note the person is unresponsive to a particular foreplay activity, move on to another. If the person remains unresponsive to all your foreplay efforts, try returning to initialization/seduction mode.

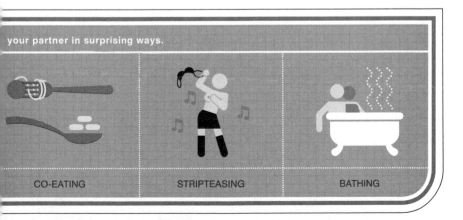

your partner in surprising ways.

CO-EATING   STRIPTEASING   BATHING

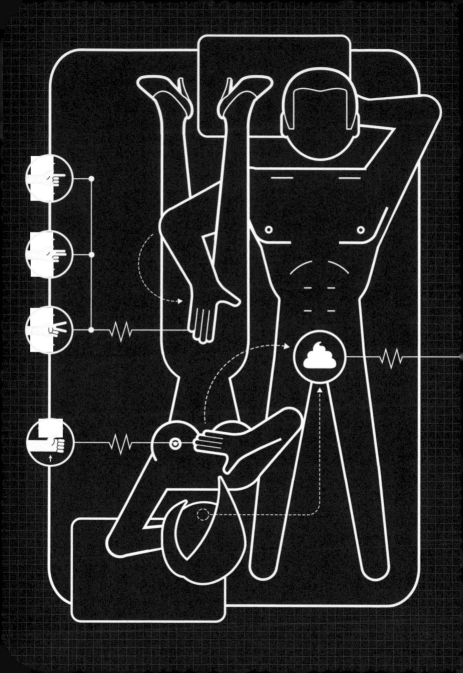

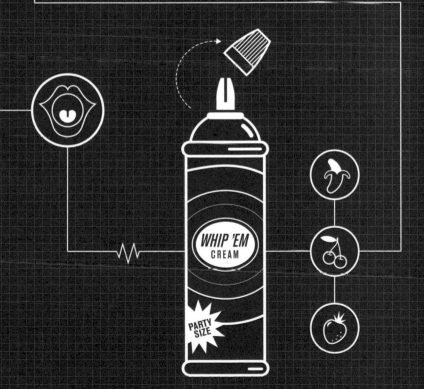

[Chapter 3]

Manual and Oral Genital Operation

The male and female genitalia represent the focal point of sexual activity. Designed for coupling in full genital interface, genitals can also be operated in many gratifying nonintercourse activities. Servicing the genitals with your hands and other parts of your body can lead to great pleasure and even sexual climax—and/or prepare them for full genital interface. Remember that attitude is nearly as important as technique when operating the genitals. The object of your attention wants to feel that you are respectful and stimulating yourself while stimulating their genitalia. So approach the process with care, enthusiasm, and no small amount of reverence.

Male Genitals

The male genitals serve as the male's main sexual pleasure center, offering an opportunity for a wide variety of rewarding activities. The term penis is often used to refer to all the parts of the male genitals. But in fact the penis encompasses only the genitals' shaft and glans, plus parts like the frenulum contained on and within them. The penis plugs into the female genitals during intercourse, leading to potentially great pleasure for both persons. It also dispenses the genetic fluid necessary for reproduction. It is available in two basic styles: circumcised and uncircumcised.

Diagram and Parts List

Size and proportions will vary. However, each set of male genitals usually comes with the following preinstalled sexual features. If one or more of these parts are missing or malfunctioning, contact an authorized service provider immediately.

Foreskin (uncircumcised models only): This sleeve of flesh covers the head of the genitals. It contains "smart sensors" that conduct pleasure and aid in regulating arousal levels. The foreskin is surgically removed shortly after birth on circumcised models, leaving an exposed glans.

⚠️ *WARNING: Circumcision has become a flashpoint for debate in recent years, with some men claiming that removal of the foreskin adversely impacts sexual sensitivity. Some have even taken the radical step of having "corrective" surgery—so-called foreskin restoration or reverse circumcision—which involves stretching and/or taping the skin around the glans to create an artificial foreskin. However, the actual foreskin and its functions can never be fully recovered since the natural foreskin contains special nerve endings and blood vessels that make its inherent functions possible.*

Glans: The bulb-shaped head, or glans, sits at the end of the shaft (and beneath the foreskin on uncircumcised models). Rich with nerve endings, it can provide intense pleasure when properly stimulated. Due to its soft, spongy texture and ergonomic design, the glans also cushions and stimulates the female during intercourse.

Urethra: This small opening at the tip of the glans works as a dispensing portal for genetic fluid, or semen, and is highly sensitive.

Shaft: This complex hydraulic mechanism contains cylinders filled with small blood vessels. During periods of stimulation, blood flows into these cylinders, causing the genitals to stiffen and swell. This enlarged state and erect posture signals that the male is prepared for full interface mode.

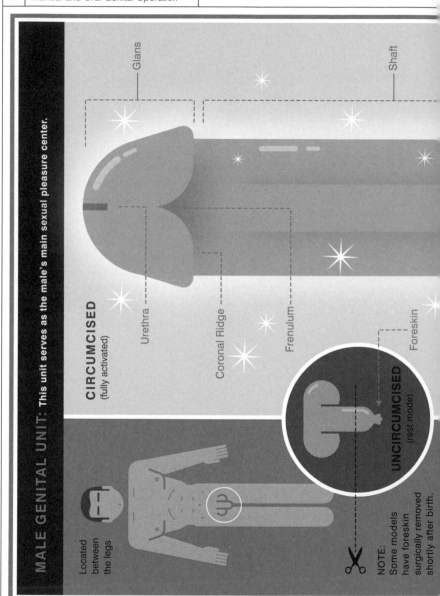

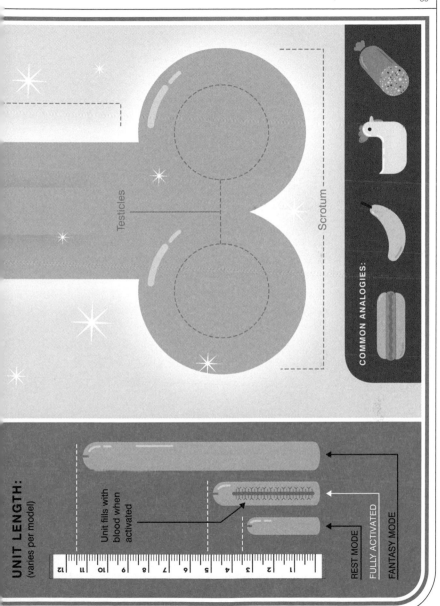

UNIT LENGTH:
(varies per model)

Unit fills with blood when activated

REST MODE

FULLY ACTIVATED

FANTASY MODE

Testicles

Scrotum

COMMON ANALOGIES:

Frenulum: This web of tissues connects the foreskin to the underside of the glans on uncircumcised models. It remains intact on most circumcised models. It looks like a small break on the underside of the glans. Densely laden with nerve endings, it is an extremely sensitive pleasure spot.

Coronal Ridge: The coronal ridge forms a rim between the glans and shaft. When properly stimulated, it can work in tandem with the frenulum to inspire the male to peak performance.

Scrotum: Attached to the bottom of the shaft, this soft sack contains dual pouches that house the testicles. These pouches operate as semen-production and storage centers. The testicles also produce testosterone, the main male sexual hormone, which helps inspire males to engage in interface mode. These orb-shaped items can also be stimulated for pleasure.

Pubic Hair: Fine and curly on most persons, pubic hair covers much of the area on and around the male genitals, excluding the glans and much of the shaft.

Length: The average male genitals measure 3.5 by 1.25 inches (8.9 x 3.2 cm) in rest mode and 5.1 by 1.6 inches (13 x 4 cm) when fully activated. Sizes and perception of sizes vary widely.

⚠ **WARNING:** *Male genital enlargement, sometimes called "penile enhancement," has become something of a cottage industry in recent decades. Methods designed to increase the length and girth of the male member include inflatable implants, vacuum pumps, herbal supplements, and phalloplasty, or penile surgery. Stretching of the male genitals through the use of hanging extenders and weights is also quite popular. The efficacy of these techniques is open*

to debate, however, and ample evidence exists to suggest that many such practices do more harm than good. It is wise to subject all claims of genital enhancement—especially those involving clamps and weights—to the same scrutiny
and skepticism one would apply to any radical surgical procedure.

Unit Curvature

Some females (and many males) grow alarmed at the sight of a curved
penis. However, neither the straightness of the penis nor the angle at which
an erection juts out from the pelvis (commonly known as "the angle of the
dangle") has any impact upon sexual performance. In the vast majority of
cases, penis curvature is normal and just part of standard human deviation.
In rare cases, the curve is pronounced and may reflect an abnormality.
Peyronie's disease, also known as "bent nail syndrome," is a severe curvature of the penis that affects about 4 percent of males worldwide. It is distin-
guished from everyday benign curvature of the penis by the agonizing pain
and sexual dysfunction experienced by Peyronie's sufferers as a result of
their pronounced penile bend.

Unit Malfunction

Males can use this handy cheat sheet to determine if they suffer from one
of these common forms of genital malfunction.

Micropenis is a medical term used to describe an abnormally small penis.
Estimates vary as to the worldwide incidence of micropenis, which may
stem from pubescent hormone deficiency. It is often treated with a combi-
nation of phalloplasty and testosterone injections.

Phimosis derives its name from the Greek word for "muzzle." Muzzle is a
word no man wants to have associated with his penis. Millions of adults

worldwide are afflicted with this maddening condition, in which the foreskin of the penis cannot be retracted, thus inhibiting normal penile function.

Hypospadias. Is your urethral meatus in the wrong place? If you even understand that question, chances are you suffer from hypospadias, a condition that afflicts one in every 125 infant males. Put most bluntly, hypospadias is a misplaced pee hole. The tiny hole, known as the urethral meatus, may be set back far down the penile shaft. In severe cases, sexual function may be impossible.

Priapism. If your doctor told you that you were priapic, you might normally take it as a compliment. Priapus, after all, was the Greek god of fertility, recognizable in statuary by his enormous genitalia. But the medical condition named after him is nothing to boast about. Clinical priapism is a prolonged, often painful erection that is not associated with sexual stimulation. Imagine walking around all day in this agonizing and embarrassing state. It's no secret that a lot of men would be afraid to discuss this condition openly.

Female Genitals

The female genitals operate as the female's main sexual pleasure center, offering a wide variety of rewarding foreplay and intercourse activities. It serves as a "modem" for the male genitals to plug into during full interface, leading to potentially great pleasure for both persons as well as the reception of genetic fluid for reproduction.

⚠ *EXPERT TIP: The terms vulva and vagina are often used independently to refer to all the parts of the female genitals. In fact, the vulva encompasses only the genitals' exterior elements, and the vagina is technically the internal corridor leading from the vulva to the uterus.*

Diagram and Parts List

Size and proportions vary. However, each set of female genitals usually comes with the following preinstalled sexual features. If one or more parts are missing or malfunctioning, contact an authorized service provider immediately.

Labia Majora (Outer Lips): The labia majora consist of two thick vertical lips that stretch from the mons to the bottom of the vulva. The outer portion of each lip is usually covered with hair, whereas the inner side is smooth. The rest of the external and internal parts of the female genitals lie within the labia majora.

Labia Minora (Inner Lips): These thinner vertical lips rest inside the labia majora and surround the rest of the vulva and its parts.

Clitoral Hood: Positioned at the top of the labia minora, the clitoral hood forms a protective cap over the clitoris.

FEMALE GENITAL UNIT: This serves as the female's main pleasure center.

COMMON ANALOGIES

mons
clitoris
clitoral hood
labia majora
urethra
vagina
hymen
labia minora
anus
g-spot
cervix

Clitoris: Thickly packed with nerve endings, the clitoris is the most sensitive and erotically charged part of the female anatomy. Consisting of a shaft and head, the clitoris appears for only about an inch outside the body. The rest of the clitoris extends internally.

⚠ **EXPERT TIP:** *Some people have claimed that the clitoris is the only body part designed entirely for pleasure. However, this claim is incorrect. In fact, when stimulated, the clitoris swells and closes the urethra to harmful bacteria, thus helping to prevent bladder infection.*

Urethra: This tube serves as the output point for urine and, if properly stimulated, can also be a source of pleasure.

⚠ **WARNING:** *Internal urethral stimulation can cause serious harm. Limit stimulation to massage of the outside area.*

Mons: Although not technically part of the vulva, this round mound of flesh sits just above the vulva and is usually covered with pubic hair.

Pubic Hair: Fine and curly on most models, pubic hair covers the mons and other parts of the vulva. It usually grows in a shape roughly like an upside-down triangle (occasionally referred to as "the Dorito"), but many persons, both male and female alike, reshape their pubic hair into different "hairstyles" through cutting, shaving, and waxing.

Internal Affairs

With female genitalia, there is a little more than meets the eye. Here is a closer look at the inner workings of the female anatomy.

Vagina: Beginning at an opening within the labia minora just below the urethra, the vagina is a corridor that extends into the cervix, or gate to the womb. In rest mode, the average vagina extends about four inches (10 cm) in length and one inch (2.5 cm) in diameter. It lengthens, widens, and self-lubricates as the female becomes erotically activated. Once activated, the vagina can expand or contract to snugly accommodate male genitalia of almost any size.

Hymen: A small crescent-shaped membrane at the vaginal opening that tears and disappears during the first introduction of male genitalia into the vagina. Often considered a symbol of virginity, the hymen can also tear during heavy exercise, stretching, or other stress to the area.

G-spot: A small band of raised nerves about the size of a quarter situated on the front wall of the vagina a few inches inside the vaginal opening. Like the external clitoris, the internal G-spot can, if properly stimulated, bring about sexual climax.

EXPERT TIP: Named for the German gynecologist Ernst Gräfenberg, who first "discovered" it, the G-spot is considered to be a critical component in a woman's ability to experience vaginal orgasm. Sexologists continue to debate its role in fostering female ejaculation, also known as "gushing."

Cervix: A cone-shaped entryway at the back of the vagina that marks the beginning of the uterus. A male who can penetrate a woman deeply enough that he can feel her cervix with his penis is said to have "hit bottom." Doing so often causes discomfort for the female.

PUBIC FLAIR: Sporting a new pubic hairstyle can enhance one's appearance.

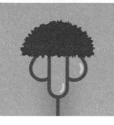

THE NATURAL:
Thick and bushy

THE HEART:
Trimmed into a heart shape

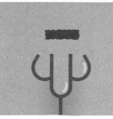

THE HITLERSTACHE:
The groin area is shaved except area above groin

SMILEY FACE:
Rounded top with eyes and mouth shaved in

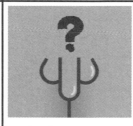

QUESTION MARK:
Line curled at top, with dot on bottom

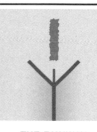

THE RUNWAY:
Thin vertical strip (AKA the Landing Strip)

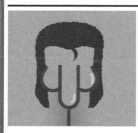

THE ELVIS:
Bushy on top, bare in the middle, and "sideburns" on either flank

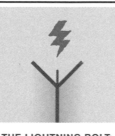

THE LIGHTNING BOLT:
A jagged line shaved at an angle

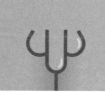

THE BALDY:
All hair removed

Lubrication

Moistening of the genitals, both male and female, with a slippery sub-stance to reduce friction and increase pleasure is essential prior to most genital sexual activities. Too little lubrication can lead to discom-fort or injury as well as the tearing of condoms or other protective devices. Most females will lubricate naturally when properly stimulated, though applying additional lubricant remains a wise precaution. Male genitals require the application of lubricant prior to manual stimulation or intercourse.

Saliva can provide a serviceable lubricant. A sufficient supply is often spread over the genitals during oral-sex operations. A variety of prefabricated lubricants, available from most drug, grocery, and con-venience stores, come in these basic varieties:

Oil-Based: Once the standard, oil-based lubes have fallen out of favor in recent years due to their tendency to degrade condoms and other protec-tive devices. They are also difficult to wash off clothes and bedding and often leave a permanent stain. They remain in the vagina long after sex and lead to infections and other health problems.

Water-Based: Smoother and slicker than their oil-based counterparts, water-based lubricants easily clean off bedding, clothing, and the skin with a wet washcloth. They will not corrode condoms or other protective devices during sex. Water-based lubes do tend to deplete quickly during sexual activity and often need to be reapplied.

⚠ *WARNING: Many water-based lubricants contain glycerin, which can antagonize internal infections, such as yeast, in the vagina. Look for a water-based lube that is glycerin-free.*

Silicone-Based: Less thick than oil-based products, silicone lubes usually require only a single application of a thin layer throughout a full sex session. They will not come off in water, making them valuable for encounters in pools, hot tubs, or lakes. They are, however, more difficult to clean off, though not as hard as cleaning up an oil-based lube.

Specialty Lubricants: These include heating lubricants (designed to warm when applied and rubbed, adding a new layer of sensation to the intercourse experience), flavored lubricants (which are safe to ingest), and desensitizing lubricants (these desensitize the male genitals to mute stimulation and delay climax).

⚠ **EXPERT TIP:** *Spermicidal lubricants kill sperm on contact. They can provide an extra layer of protection from unwanted pregnancy during intercourse, but they are by no means foolproof. Always use a condom or other protective device to prevent the spread of disease and to avoid undesired pregnancy.*

Applying Lubricant

[**1**] Place the lubricant in a convenient and discreet place prior to the initiation of foreplay activities so that you do not have to search or fumble when it comes time to apply.

[**2**] Unless the variety is edible, do not apply the lubricant to a body part that you may place in your mouth during the rest of the interface session. For example, wait until after you have completed oral sex before applying the lubricant to the person's genitals.

[3] Spread the lubricant from its container onto your hand, then apply onto your partner's genitalia. Massage the genitalia to spread the lubricant evenly and completely.

EXPERT TIP: Apply the lubricant in a playful manner that further activates both parties' arousal. Make the process part of foreplay, not an interruption of it.

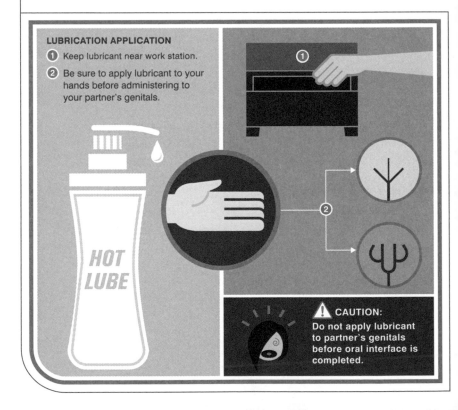

LUBRICATION APPLICATION

1. Keep lubricant near work station.
2. Be sure to apply lubricant to your hands before administering to your partner's genitals.

HOT LUBE

CAUTION: Do not apply lubricant to partner's genitals before oral interface is completed.

[4] When using the lubricant during intercourse, apply to both sets of genitals. This will increase pleasure and decrease the time necessary for the lubricant to spread from one set of genitals to the other.

[5] Keep the lubricant nearby in case reapplication is necessary.

[6] Maintain a backup supply.

[7] Immediately after the close of the intercourse session, use a warm, wet towel to clean off lubricant from both genitalia, surrounding skin, and any bedding or clothing it may have spread onto.

Manual Male Genitalia Manipulation

A highly skilled and sensitive piece of hardware, the human hand is capable of numerous activities to stimulate the penis in preparation for full interface or even for climax.

It is important to find a good position, in relation to your partner, before attempting manual manipulation of genitalia. Good positioning will make manipulation activities more efficient and rewarding and help prevent discomfort or injury caused by prolonged periods of awkward bending of the arms and neck into unnatural positions. See the charts showing possible positions for each type of stimulation at the beginning of subsequent sections.

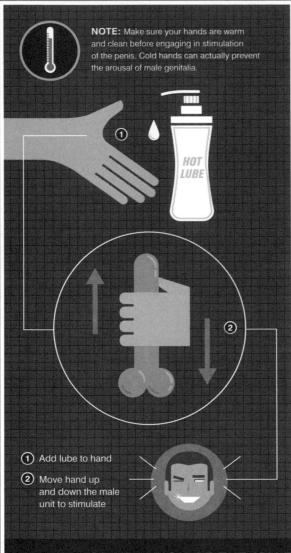

NOTE: Make sure your hands are warm and clean before engaging in stimulation of the penis. Cold hands can actually prevent the arousal of male genitalia.

HOT LUBE

(1) Add lube to hand

(2) Move hand up and down the male unit to stimulate

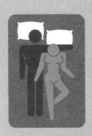

BESIDE

He lies on bed, partner lies next to him in same direction, propped on one elbow while reaching over with other hand.

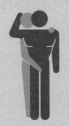

FROM BEHIND
(standing)

He stands, partner stands behind and reaches around.

MANUAL STIMULATION OF THE MALE GENITALS: **The hand**

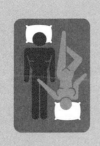

BESIDE (in other direction)

He lies on bed, partner lies next to him in opposite direction, propped on one elbow while reaching over with other hand.

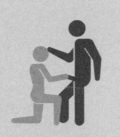

BELOW

He stands, partner kneels or crouches in front and reaches up.

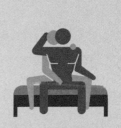

FROM BEHIND (sitting)

He sits on bed between partner's open legs, partner reaches around to his genitals.

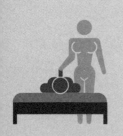

OVER TOP

Partner stands in front of bed or table that male is lying on and reaches down to touch genitals.

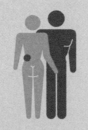

STANDING

He stands, partner stands next to and reaches down.

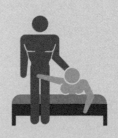

STANDING-LYING

He stands next to bed or couch that partner is lying on, partner reaches over.

can be used to stimulate the penis in preparation for full interface or even for climax.

Achieving Full Genital Activation

Many male genitals will arrive fully erect when removed from their packaging. Some with be partially erect, and others will remain flaccid and deactivated. To fully activate the genitals for servicing, try these activities.

EXPERT TIP: Using two hands enhances the effect of most of these exercises described below.

Encircling: Place the palm and fingers of one hand over the shaft and scrotum and squeeze very gently. Put your fingers beneath the scrotum and gently pull it upward. Performed while the male is still clothed, this maneuver will communicate your intention to manipulate his penis and help it become fully stimulated. It can also prove effective once the penis has been removed from its wrapping.

Lap Dancing: While the male is still dressed and seated on a sturdy chair, straddle his legs and position your buttocks over his groin area. Lower your bottom so that it brushes the top of the male's groin. Move it gently back and forth, then in circular motions. Increase the speed and pressure of your contact as you continue.

WARNING: Suddenly sitting with all your weight upon the lap of an aroused male could cause serious injury to his swollen genitals. Be wary of how much pressure you apply to this delicate area.

Puffing: Expel bursts of air through your mouth over the penis and scrotum. Try long and short puffs and moving your mouth up and down the genital area as you perform this activity. (Note: This action does not constitute what is commonly known as a "blow job" and could lead to ridicule if you perform it in response to a request for one from a male. For information on what does constitute a "blow job," see "Oral Interface with the Male Genitals," page 86.)

Hair Tickling: If your hair is long enough, dip your head so that the ends of its strands fall over the genital area and move it back and forth and in a circular manner so that it tickles the genitals. Make sure your hair is free of berets, bobby pins, curlers, or any other items that might cause injury or discomfort.

Grasp and Release: Gently grasp the base of the shaft, then release it after a few seconds. Repeat, moving up and down the penis and scrotum.

⚠ **WARNING:** *Watch for signs of arousal and approaching climax. A prematurely "popped cork" can dampen sexual activity before it can be properly said to have started. If you do not want the male to reach climax during these activities, communicate with him to find out if he is nearing ejaculation so that you can adjust your approach.*

Bouncing: Grasp the base of the shaft and wiggle your wrist so that the glans and top of the shaft bounces up and down. Move your hand in a circular motion so the glans draws an "O" in the air.

Tickling: Glide your moistened index finger around the glans and up and down the frenulum on the underside of the glans.

Ironing: Place your palm against the underside of the shaft and press it toward the male's stomach. Glide your palm from the base of the shaft to the glans as you continue to gently apply downward pressure. Use both hands, placing one on either side of the shaft. For added effect, bend forward as you move your hands up the shaft so that your breasts brush against the shaft and glans as your hands move to the top of the shaft and head.

Polishing: With a generous amount of lube or saliva on your palm, move it up and down the shaft, over the head, and across and underneath the scrotum, as if you were polishing them.

EXPERT TIP: *The perineum, a small band between the bottom of the scrotum and the anus, is highly sensitive. Many men enjoy having this area gently stroked with lubricated fingertips.*

Fluttering: Brush the fingertips of both hands up and down the shaft and over the glans.

Shimmying: Grasp the base of the penis, then move your hand up the shaft and over the head. Repeat.

Doorknobbing: Grasp the shaft of the penis with one hand. Turn your other hand downward so that its thumb and fingers hang like vines. Now place them around the head of the penis. Gently twirl them around the head as if you were trying to gently turn a doorknob.

EXPERT TIP: *If the male indicates that he is about to orgasm and you want to prevent it, firmly squeeze the base of his penis and push the head gently toward his scrotum. Hold until his urge to climax passes.*

Shutdown Mode

The following exercises take the stimulation of the male genitals to the next level and can sometimes bring about an orgasm.

Hand over Hand: Softly encircle the glans with one hand then move it slowly and gently down the shaft. Once that hand reaches the base, encircle the glans with your other hand and perform the same motion. Repeat, one hand after the other, alternating the speed and amount of pressure.

Ringing: Join the tips of your thumb and index finger into a circle around the top of the penis and move them up and down the shaft. Twist your wrist as you move to vary and intensify the sensations.

Rubbing: Place each palm on opposite sides of the shaft. Move them up and down the shaft as you gently push them toward each other, as if you were rubbing them together to warm them up.

EXPERT TIP: Occasionally look into the male's eyes as you perform these exercises. Many males find a confident gaze from their partner to be highly stimulating as she manipulates his genitals. Looking into his eyes will also allow you to audit his responses to your manipulation efforts and adjust as necessary.

Reverser: Position your hand so that the thumb is pointing downward. Grasp the base of the penis with your thumb and index finger while wrapping your other three fingers around the shaft just above. Move your hand up and down, applying the greatest amount of pressure with your thumb and forefinger. By applying the most intense pressure at the bottom with your thumb and forefinger, you are creating the closest sensation to the penis sliding in and out of the vagina, which is tightest at its opening.

Cleavaging: A female with large breasts can position the penis between her breasts, then push her breasts together so that they "sandwich" the penis while moving her torso up and down so that the penis pistons between the soft folds of her breasts.

The Finisher: Wrap both hands around the shaft of the penis and move them quickly up and down the shaft and over the top of the head. Twist your hands in opposite directions as you perform the maneuver, varying your pace and the firmness of your grip.

⚠ **WARNING:** *Male sexual climax is accompanied by the spurting of a white, sticky substance, known as semen, out the urethra. The semen may shoot up to several feet from the penis head and be expelled in multiple*

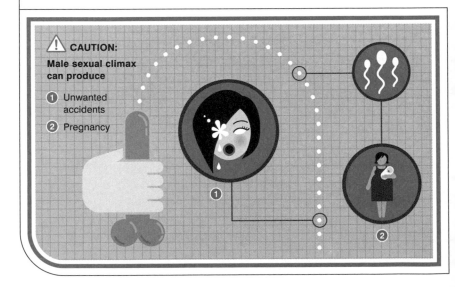

⚠ **CAUTION:**
Male sexual climax can produce

1 Unwanted accidents

2 Pregnancy

spurts. Be prepared for this event and make sure no valuable materials are in range, such as photographs, silk clothing, or other items that could be permanently stained by the semen. Keep a small towel or washcloth nearby while performing hand manipulation on the penis for quick and easy cleanup of emitted sperm. Make sure to clean the ejaculate off any surfaces, including the skin, before it dries and becomes more difficult to remove. Also, be aware that there is a period of downtime associated with male climax during which the male may be incapable of attaining another erection. The duration of this "refractory period" varies from male to male, although younger males tend to "bounce back" faster than older ones. Plan activities for this period that do not involve aroused genitalia. It may be a good time to focus on the woman's pleasure, for example. Cuddling, spooning, or even a quick game of gin rummy can help bridge the gap between erections in fine fashion.

Manual Female Genitalia Manipulation

Because they are largely hidden from plain sight, female genitalia can seem more mysterious and difficult to operate than male genitalia. But with practice, patience, and feedback, you can learn to easily stimulate the female to achieve full arousal and even climax.

Unlike male genitalia, the vagina instantly reloads after climax. It can continue to receive attention and often achieve several more climaxes. So you will not have to stop short of bringing the female to orgasm for fear that she will be spent for further activities.

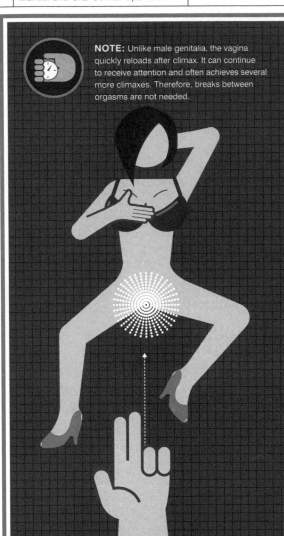

NOTE: Unlike male genitalia, the vagina quickly reloads after climax. It can continue to receive attention and often achieves several more climaxes. Therefore, breaks between orgasms are not needed.

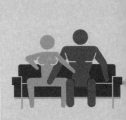

BESIDE (sitting)

She sits on couch, partner sits beside her and reaches over and down.

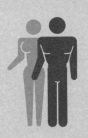

IN FRONT (standing)

She stands, partner stands in front and slightly to side while reaching down.

MANUAL STIMULATION OF THE FEMALE GENITALS: With practice

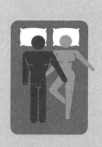

BESIDE (lying)

She lies on bed, partner lies beside her in same direction, propped on one elbow and reaching over.

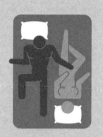

BESIDE (lying in other direction)

She lies on bed, partner lies next to her with head facing other direction, reaches over.

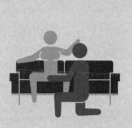

IN FRONT (sitting)

She sits on couch, partner kneels or crouches between her open legs and reaches up.

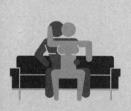

FROM BEHIND (sitting)

She sits on couch, partner sits behind, with legs on either side of her, and reaches around.

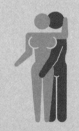

FROM BEHIND (standing)

She stands, partner stands behind and reaches around.

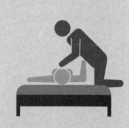

OVER TOP, TO SIDE

She lies on bed or couch, partner stands on side at approximately 90 degrees and reaches down.

patience, and feedback, you can learn to stimulate the female to full arousal and even climax.

Achieving Full Genital Activation

Most female genitals require more time and attention than male genitals to become fully prepared for vigorous sexual activities. When fully activated, parts of the female genitals will swell with blood, though not as dramatically as the male genitals. They will also moisten, making interface more expedient and pleasurable. To fully activate the genitals for servicing, try these activities.

Upper Leg Rubbing: Stroke the sensitive flesh on her inner thighs. Tickle the back of her knee, then gently move upward toward her genitals. Alternate the pace and pressure, using your palm or fingertips. Dance your fingertips up and down the inner thigh. Try with both hands, one on each leg.

Mons Rubbing: Place your palm on her mons, the mound of soft flesh just above the vulva. Rub gently in a circular motion. Push gently downward. Let your fingers fall over her genitals.

Labia Dancing: Dance your fingertips lightly over the outer labia lips.

EXPERT TIP: *For heightened arousal, continue kissing and/or performing breast manipulation with your mouth and free hand while engaging in vaginal stimulation activities.*

External Massage: Place your thumbs and fingers on the opposite side of her genitals at the bottom of the outside of her outer labia lips. Move them upward, massaging the skin just outside her genital area.

Deep Massage: Grasp the outer labia lips of her vagina with your fingers. Gently twist and knead them up and down, sometimes in synch, sometimes in opposite directions, so that they rub against each other. This is the one vaginal maneuver you can perform with relative vigor and pressure without causing pain or injury. Still, proceed gently at first, gradually building up pace and pressure.

EXPERT TIP: If the female is unresponsive to your efforts, ask her for advice on how best to stimulate her genitals. Or ask her to do it with her own hand while you watch, or place your hand on top of hers as she performs self-stimulation.

The Pinch: Slowly pull the outer lips out and up, then roll them back down over the clitoral hood. Repeat.

Airing: Place each thumb on either side of the outer labia and push them outward in opposite directions, parting her outer lips and exposing her inner labia lips. Let the outer lips fall back together and repeat.

EXPERT TIP: If your activation efforts continue to be unsuccessful, place your hand over her vagina area and let her grind against it in a way that activates her.

Shutdown Mode

The following exercises take the stimulation of the female genitals to the next level and can sometimes bring about an orgasm. Keep in mind that female genitalia are much more sensitive and fragile than those of the male. A positive response from the female to your genital manipu-lation efforts does not mean that you should press harder or faster—unless she specifically asks you to go faster and harder. Just maintain

the same approximate pace and firmness, alternating subtly, and, as always, watch for responses from your partner.

Tapping: Gently tap the clitoral hood with your palm or fingertips. Repeat at the speed and pressure that pleases her most.

Gentle Grasping: Grasp the clitoral hood softly between your thumb and index finger. Lightly rub the two sides of it together so the inner sides of the hood brush against the clitoris.

Light Touching: Part the clitoral hood and very lightly trace your finger over the clitoris. The rule on direct clitoral stimulation is, the lighter the touch, the more stimulating the action.

Vaginal Stimulation: Place your index or middle finger slowly and gently into her vaginal opening. Make sure she is sufficiently stimulated and naturally lubricated before proceeding. If not, apply lube to your finger. Circle your finger slowly around the inside. Slowly move the finger deeper.

G-Spot Stimulation: Once the finger is completely inside, flick it back toward the front stomach-side of the vaginal wall. You should feel a spongy, slightly raised mound about the size of a quarter a few inches inside. This is the female G-spot, a highly sensitive erotic area. Continue flicking your finger back and forth so that the underside of its tip bounces gently off and rubs against the G-spot. This maneuver will bring many women quickly to orgasm.

⚠ *WARNING: The clitoris is an incredibly sensitive apparatus and, thus, prone to irritation and injury if you manipulate it too vigorously or without enough lubricant. Many women shy away from the intensity of direct clitoral stimulation and prefer the sensation of the clitoral hood rubbing against it. If you do make direct contact, do so as lightly as possible. A soft touch will not only prevent discomfort but will also prove more stimulating for the vast majority of females. Also, always make sure your fingers are sufficiently lubricated before directly touching the clitoris.*

Oral Genital Operation

Due to its intimacy and the high potential for inducing orgasm, oral-genital interface can serve as both a preparation for full genital interface as well as a highly satisfying alternative.

Since the genitals also act as a urine dispenser and spend most of their day packaged in a dark, sweaty, and sometimes malodorous place, they will usually require thorough hygienic maintenance before being suitable for oral attention. Make sure your partner's genitals receive a fresh washing prior to oral servicing. When preparing any genitals for oral servicing, be sure to deodorize them with soap, then rinse them thoroughly to remove all soap or synthetic lubricant residue left over from manual activation activities; you do not want these substances to end up in your or your partner's mouth. Also, remember to cleanse the anus, which sits within inches of the bottom of the genitals and can aromatically intrude on oral servicing activities.

One enjoyable option is to take a bath, shower, or dip in a hot tub together just before oral sex. This activity will cleanse both sets of genitals and allow each partner to engage in additional foreplay activities, which can be extra stimulating in or beneath warm water.

Oral Interface with the Male Genitals

Attitude is nearly as important as technique in the oral servicing of male genitalia, a process commonly known as fellatio, or a "blow job." If the male senses that the female is bored and simply going through the motions, he will enjoy the experience far less and may even suffer a full sexual-system shutdown. Approach these activities with enthusiasm and respect.

Initialization

The most effective way to inspire the male to orgasm is by simultaneously performing a manual- and oral-interface exercise on his genitals. Successful oral interface should include stroking, using a hand, and the exploration of testicles, thighs, and possibly the anal region. Test out different combinations to see which one works best for your partner. Keeping teeth covered by the lips is essential. However, occasional nibbling on the genitals is an option. Just make sure that this action is performed very gently, and keep the nibbling to the shaft, which is less sensitive.

Rather than immediately stuffing the glans and shaft into your mouth, heighten the pleasure of oral interface for the recipient of your attentions as well as yourself by warming up with these exercises.

Kissing: Purse your lips and plant quick, gentle kisses on various parts of the genitals—the glans, shaft, scrotum, and so on.

Frenulum Licking: Lightly trace your tongue along the highly sensitive frenulum located on the underside of the glans. Most males prefer an upward motion.

Butterflying: Flutter the tip of your tongue around the top of the glans, then around its coronal ridge. Swirl it in one direction, then the other.

Lick over the top of the glans to the coronal ridge on one side, across half the coronal ridge, then back across the glans to the coronal ridge on the other side. If he is uncircumcised, you first need to gently pull his foreskin downward to expose the glans before performing this or any other glans-stimulation exercises.

Scrotum Play: Lick the underside of the scrotum. Take one testicle in your mouth and gently suck. Repeat on the other testicle. Do not bite down on the testicles, as this may cause excruciating pain.

EXPERT TIP: If you are concerned about the transmission of bodily fluids, and the attendant risk of sexually transmitted diseases, consider using a condom for oral sex. Make sure to use an unlubricated variety that doesn't contain a spermicide. There are many flavored condoms on the market, ranging from chocolate to banana. Just make sure your brand is sugar-free and FDA-approved for strength and protection.

Variations

Many couples use oral manipulation as a means to fully activate the male genitals for intercourse. Most males can climax only once without needing to recuperate for at least a half hour, often much longer. Avoid overstimulation of the male genitals if you wish to employ them in genital interface soon thereafter.

If the goal of the oral interface is to bring the male to orgasm, however, these exercises will provide a more vigorous and efficient form of stimulation. Remember to vary your technique. Stick with one for a minute or a few seconds only, then move on to another. The variety will heighten the sensation and also help jaw and neck muscles from growing sore or cramped from staying too long in one position. Identify the technique that seems to

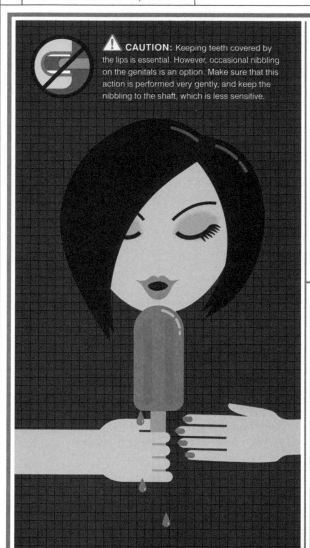

CAUTION: Keeping teeth covered by the lips is essential. However, occasional nibbling on the genitals is an option. Make sure that this action is performed very gently, and keep the nibbling to the shaft, which is less sensitive.

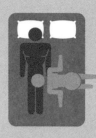

BESIDE (lying)

He lies on couch or mattress, partner props self on one elbow and leans over.

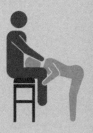

STANDING OVERTOP, TO FRONT

He sits on high table or countertop, partner stands in front and leans down.

ORAL STIMULATION OF THE MALE GENITALS: Attitude is

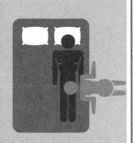

BESIDE (kneeling)

He lies on couch, partner kneels on floor next to couch and leans over.

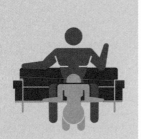

IN FRONT

He sits on chair, partner kneels between his open legs.

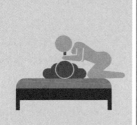

STANDING OVERTOP, TO SIDE

He lies on bed, partner stands on side of bed and leans down.

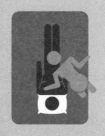

SIDE BY SIDE

He lies in one direction on bed, partner lies in the other direction, with head in front of his genitals.

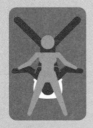

"69"

Partners lie in opposite directions, with each head positioned in front of partner's genitals.

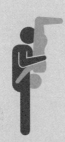

STANDING "69"

He stands, holding partner upside-down so partner's genitals are in his face and partner's face is in front of his genitals.

nearly as important as technique in the oral servicing of male genitalia.

give your partner the most pleasure and return to it when you want to bring him quickly to climax.

■ Place the glans in your mouth and alternate between gently sucking it and moving your tongue over and around it.
■ Cover your teeth with your lips and encircle the glans with your mouth. Then move your lips down to the shaft. Slowly piston your lips up and down the shaft, alternating speeds and the amount of pressure you apply with your mouth. You can apply more pressure to the shaft than other parts of the genitals, but be sure not to press on it too hard with your lips.
■ Stimulate the glans with the roof of your mouth as you massage the shaft with your lips. Simultaneously use your tongue to tickle the shaft and glans.

EXPERT TIP: *Many males find varying temperatures on their genitals highly stimulating. Keep a glass of ice water nearby. Rub an ice cube on your lips before performing oral genital manipulation. Rub the ice cube up and down the shaft, then use your warm mouth on it, rubbing it again with the ice cube. With practice using a small, smooth ice cube, you can keep the cube in your mouth as you orally manipulate the male genitals, leading to a constant variation of hot and cold on the unit.*

Semen Management

Male genitals erupt during orgasm, shooting semen through the shaft and out the top of the glans, usually at a high rate of speed. The volume of semen will vary from person to person and climax to climax. If you have your mouth overtop of the glans and down the shaft, be prepared for the eruption so that it doesn't shoot down your throat and cause you to gag. It is also important to keep track of the semen after ejaculation so that none accidentally ends up in the vagina, which can spread sexually transmitted diseases (STDs) or may result in unwanted pregnancy. Individual sperm within the semen can live several hours, even days, and only one sperm is required to initiate a pregnancy.

Many males find it erotic for their partners to swallow the semen ejected into their mouths during oral sex, and some are even offended if their partners spit it out. While most persons find the taste and texture of semen unpleasant, they may acclimate to swallowing it and refrain from gagging. If you prefer not to, try these alternatives.

Cleavaging: As the scrotum is indicating that the male is near climax, place the glans and shaft between your breasts, moving it in and out of your cleavage. Let the ejaculate spread over your chest.

Rubbing: Finish the genital interface with your hands instead of your mouth and catch the ejaculated semen in your palms.

Smearing: After allowing the genitals to ejaculate onto your hands or breasts, erotically rub it around the breasts in view of the male. Act as if you enjoy being "marked" by his semen. Pretend to lick some from your fingertips while looking in his eyes.

Cheeking: Rub the shaft and glans next to your cheek during climax while grasping it with your hand. Let the semen run down your hands and the side of your face.

⚠ *WARNING: After orally interfacing with a male, be sure to check your hair to make sure no semen ended up tangled in the strands. Being spotted with semen in your hair can be embarrassing and will make it impossible to deny what activities you were engaged in earlier. If you find semen in your hair, encircle the affected strands with a moist washcloth and gently pull it away. Dab the spot where the semen was to make sure you removed all of it. Also, be sure to check all of your hair, since male genitals spurt several batches of semen during orgasm.*

Oral Interface with the Female Genitals

Attitude is nearly as important as technique in the oral servicing of female genitalia, a process commonly known as cunnilingus or "eating out at the Y." If the woman senses that you are uneasy or just going through the motions, she will enjoy the experience far less and may even suffer total sexual-system shutdown. Approach these activities with enthusiasm and respect. Also, don't rush through the cunnilingus process. Begin slowly, relishing the experience, and continue with care and reverence.

Many females can actually achieve orgasm more easily through oral interface than intercourse. Unlike most men, most women can orgasm multiple times with little or no rest between climaxes, so there is no need to hold back in your activation efforts, unless your partner dictates otherwise.

Initialization

Many rush straight for the clitoris during cunnilingus, but it's usually better to end up there. Stimulating other parts of the female genitals first inspires the lips to swell with blood, heightening arousal and sensitivity all over the genital area, including the clitoris.

Note that many females can experience particularly pleasurable orgasms from oral and manual servicing of their genitals through strategic delay. Use your hand and/or tongue to manipulate the female to the brink of climax, then stop. Pause for 15 seconds, then return to the activity and technique until she reaches the brink of orgasm again, then retreat to another activity. After a lengthy buildup and several stops and starts, return to the favored activity until the female achieves an orgasm. It will often prove more intense and satisfying than a normal climax. This approach can be effective with males as well.

Labia Lick: Move your tongue up and down her outer labia lips on one side, then the other. Part her outer lips with your fingers and lick her inner labia lips. Clasp her inner labia lips between your oral lips and run your tongue up and down between them.

Vaginal In and Out: Fold your tongue in two (into the shape of a taco shell) and insert it into her vaginal entry. Move it quickly in and out of her vagina. Swirl it slowly around the edges and inner walls. If you have an extraordinarily long tongue, you may be able to reach it up and around to stimulate her G-spot. But if you can't, just concentrate on the vaginal walls right inside her opening, which are rich with nerve endings.

⚠ *WARNING: Never blow into the interior of the vagina as this can cause an air embolism, a potentially deadly condition in which air bubbles travel into the bloodstream.*

Urethra: Gently trace your tongue around the entrance to the urethra.

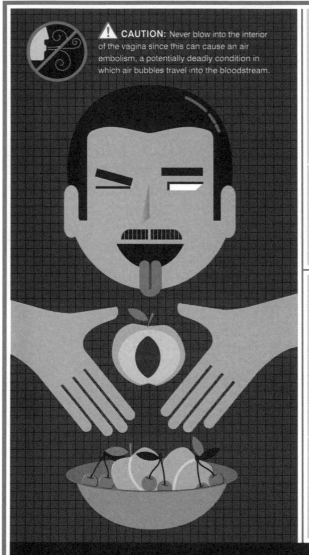

CAUTION: Never blow into the interior of the vagina since this can cause an air embolism, a potentially deadly condition in which air bubbles travel into the bloodstream.

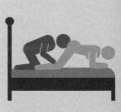

BASIC

She lies on her back on bed with legs spread, he lies on stomach with his face in her genitals.

FROM BEHIND

She lies on bed on her stomach with buttocks raised, partner kneels behind. (Variation: She stands while partner kneels behind her.)

ORAL STIMULATION OF THE FEMALE GENITALS: Attitude is

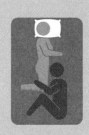

BESIDE

She lies on bed, partner lies next to her in same direction, with head at her genitals.

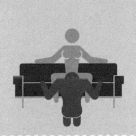

IN FRONT OF

She sits on chair, partner kneels between her open legs.

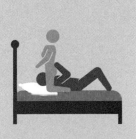

ON TOP

Partner lies on bed, she sits on top, straddling partner's face.

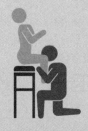

STANDING UNDERNEATH

She sits on high table or countertop, partner stands in front with face at her genitals.

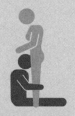

SITTING UNDERNEATH

She stands, he sits between her legs.

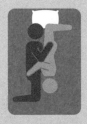

"69"

He lies in one direction, partner lies in the other with both of their heads positioned in front of partner's genitals.

nearly as important as technique in the oral servicing of female genitalia.

Variations

The clitoris is the most sensitive and erotically charged apparatus on the female body. It can be stimulated with the lightest of touches. In fact, the lighter the touch and slower the movement, the more effective the exercise will likely be. Moving too hard or too fast on the clitoris can lead to pain, total sexual-system shutdown, and even injury. In fact, many women find indirect oral stimulation of their clitorises more satisfying than direct contact.

Clitoral Hood: Lick around the clitoral hood and then take it into your mouth and gently suckle it. The hood will transmit the resulting sensations to the clitoris.

Clitoris: Part the clitoral hood with your fingers or tongue and gently touch the tip of your tongue on the clitoris. Move it slowly and lightly around the clitoral head and shaft. Draw circles, curved shapes, and cursive letters with your tongue over the clitoris. Blow lightly onto the apparatus, then repeat the exercises with your tongue. Audit the person's auditory and body language responses to your efforts and repeat the ones that get the most enthusiastic responses.

Simultaneous G-spot and Clitoral Stimulation: Simultaneous manual stimulation of the G-spot and oral stimulation of the clitoris can prove deeply satisfying to many females. Prop yourself on one elbow at a 90-degree angle from the direction the female is lying. Insert your finger into her vagina and reach up to stimulate her G-spot. Now lean over, part her clitoral hood, and stimulate her clitoris with your tongue. If performed properly, the combined stimulation of her two genital hot spots can bring about quick and deeply satisfying orgasms. Note that proper positioning and coordination can take practice, but it is well worth the effort.

⚠ **EXPERT TIP:** *If you are concerned about the transmission of bodily fluids—and the attendant risk of sexually transmitted diseases—consider employing what is known as a "dental dam," a rectangular sheet of latex used in dentistry. This flexible membrane can be purchased at most purveyors of sexual accessories and dental supply stores. To use, simply place the membrane over the vulva (or, in alternative applications, the anus) and resume normal oral stimulation of the area.*

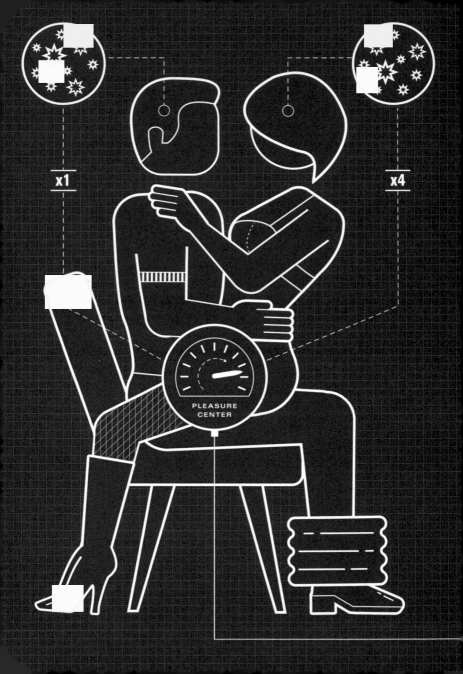

Chapter 4

Intercourse

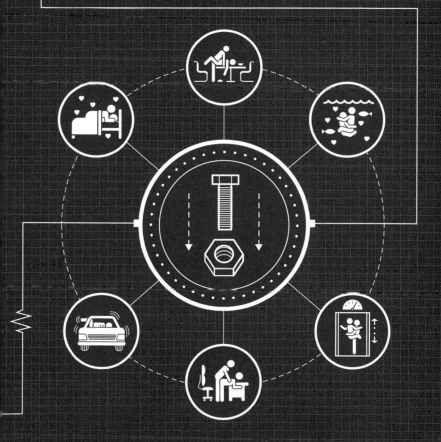

Full genital interface, or sexual intercourse, marks the climactic and often the most satisfying stage of the erotic encounter. If properly executed, intercourse can generate intense pleasure and intimacy, plus orgasms for both parties. Mismanaged, the operation can lead to physical and emotional discomfort. It can also cause the accidental generation of new persons through impregnation and represents the most efficient means of spreading sexually transmitted diseases. The activity should not be approached lightly or without preparation and knowledge.

Configuring Your Work Station

Sexual intercourse can take place in a variety of locations throughout your living quarters, and even outdoors. However, it is best to establish a special work station inside your living quarters that is especially suited for genital interface. The location should offer privacy and easy access from your final seduction station, and it should include the following items.

The Bed

The bed ranks as the most important object in your genital-interface work station. It should be appropriately sized, properly placed, stable, and comfortable.

Size: Beds come in single, double, queen, and king sizes. Larger beds such as kings and queens offer more space for movement and position options for sexual interfacing, as well as greater comfort for post-interface sleep mode. Choose the bed that best fits your needs and the space available.

Placement: For additional privacy, position the bed in an area that is remote from adjoining rooms or domiciles. A wall on at least one side will help brace the bed and keep it from migrating during vigorous intercourse activities. But make sure to leave standing room on at least two sides to facilitate certain final interface postures and maneuvers.

Stability: Test out the bed to ensure it can withstand the weight of two people engaged in vigorous interfacing activities. Bounce on it several times with your full body weight. Try standing next to the bed, coming down on it with your buttocks, standing quickly back up, and repeating. Or just bounce on top of it as though it were a trampoline. You may also wish to lock the wheels beneath its frame to ensure it remains in place. If the model you choose is not equipped with wheels and locks, place rubber pads beneath the legs of the frame to protect your floors from damage and to help stabilize the bed. Alternatively, you can push the bed against a wall or into a corner. Then be sure to direct your intercourse thrusting toward one of the walls against which it is propped.

Comfort: The thick upper layer of the bed or mattress should be firm enough to support you and another person, yet soft enough to provide a comfortable reclining area before, during, and after intercourse. Because intercourse depletes a large amount of energy, many participants transition into sleep mode shortly after its completion. Although this common post-interface activity may cause certain inconveniences, engaging in it with your partner can also perpetuate greater intimacy and increase the chances for future sexual encounters. You may even decide to reinterface shortly after waking up from sleep mode.

⚠ **WARNING:** *Waterbeds—essentially mattresses filled with water— were introduced to the mass market in the late 1960s, at the height of the sexual revolution. As a result, they came to be associated with sexual libera- tion and the "swinging" lifestyle characteristic of that era. Hugh Hefner, for example, had a king-size waterbed installed at his Playboy Mansion. In pop- ular culture, waterbeds are still occasionally portrayed as the epitome of lib- ertine chic (there is one gracing Austin Powers's bachelor pad, for instance), but they have recently come under increased scrutiny. A 2004 study by researchers at the University of Pennsylvania and Rochester University found that male waterbed users were four times more likely to be infertile than nonusers—possibly a consequence of overly warm sleeping conditions caused by the bed's heating unit.*

Other Essential Items

Sheets: Place a thin, comfortable covering, or sheet, designed to fit snugly over the mattress size of your bed. Cover that bottom fitted sheet with a top flat sheet that stretches a foot or so beyond the mattress on all sides. The fit- ted sheet protects your mattress from staining and provides comfort while you recline on it; the flat sheet helps trap body heat and keeps you warm. Consider investing in a set of high-quality bed coverings. Silk or satin sheets, or those that feature a high thread count, feel luxurious against bare skin, heightening sensual activation and making the act of getting into bed with you, and remaining there, a more appealing prospect for the other person.

Comforter or Bedspread: Cover the sheets with a thick blanket that helps warm you and the person during sleep mode or interface activities on cold days. Choose an animal print to add an extra element of wildness to your sexual encounters. Turn the boudoir into an idealized representation of the

African veldt with the addition of leopard, panther, zebra, or tiger print blanketing. Be prepared with an answer if your partner points out that there are no tigers in Africa.

Pillows: Equip the bed with pillows in a variety of shapes and sizes. These are essential as a place to rest the head during sleep mode and can be placed under body parts during intercourse to maximize stimulation in various genital interface positions. Pillows also provide a soft and pliant place to bite down during especially vigorous or intermittently painful sexual activities.

Candles: Most people prefer to interface without lamps or electric lighting devices that shine too brightly and cast light on their hardware. Candles may provide a more soothing and flattering light for final interface activities. Exercise caution when using candles: Be sure to place lit candles on a sturdy surface far enough from the bed so that they do not get knocked over during vigorous interfacing. They may set fire to the bed coverings, wall, carpet, rug, or hastily removed clothing strewn about the work station. Lamps equipped with dimmer switches and bulbs can provide a reasonable facsimile of candlelight and do not run the risk of starting a fire.

Water: Sweating during the exertion of interfacing can quickly deplete a person's liquid stores. Keep water bottles or a large pitcher of cool water with glasses near the bed to slake your thirst. Sports drinks that replenish electrolytes or specialty vitamin waters are also an option.

Recorded-Music Playing Device: As in your seduction area, this device can help set the mood and drown out sounds emanating from outside the work station. It can also help prevent those in adjacent rooms or domiciles or outside from overhearing your interface activities.

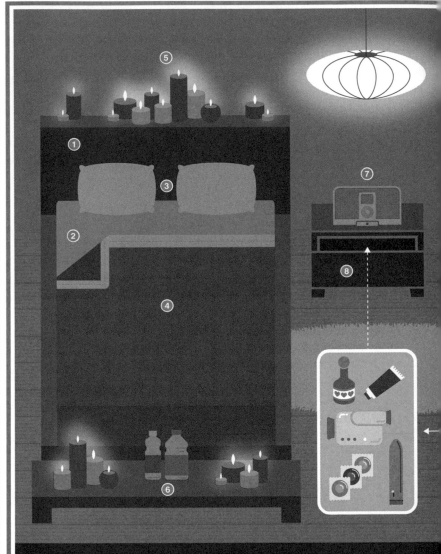

WORK STATION CONFIGURATION: A desirable work station

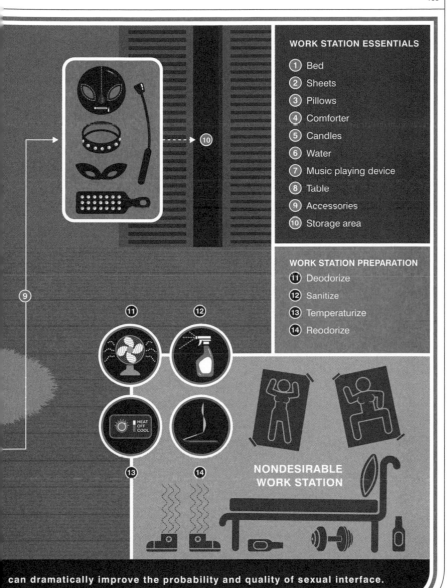

WORK STATION ESSENTIALS

1. Bed
2. Sheets
3. Pillows
4. Comforter
5. Candles
6. Water
7. Music playing device
8. Table
9. Accessories
10. Storage area

WORK STATION PREPARATION

11. Deodorize
12. Sanitize
13. Temperaturize
14. Reodorize

NONDESIRABLE WORK STATION

can dramatically improve the probability and quality of sexual interface.

Songs in the Key of Sex

Individual tastes vary, but here is a list of popular songs widely recognized as appropriate accompaniment to sexual encounters. Feel free to substitute any song that puts you and your partner in an amorous mood, fills you with sexual confidence, or approximates the rhythms you expect to achieve in your sexual encounter. Keep a CD near your bed or program your portable music device with a playlist that can be easily accessed for playback before, during, and after sexual interface.

■ "Let's Talk About Sex" by Salt-N-Pepa ■ "I Want to Fall in Love" by Chris Isaac ■ "Wild Thing" by Peaches ■ "You Sexy Thing" by Hot Chocolate ■ "Lay Lady Lay" by Bob Dylan ■ "My Humps" by The Black Eyed Peas ■ "By Your Side" by Sade ■ "Turn Me On" by Norah Jones ■ "Your Body Is a Wonderland" by John Mayer ■ "Falling Slowly" by Glen Hasard and Marketa Irglova ■ "Let's Get It On" by Marvin Gaye ■ "Sexual Healing" by Marvin Gaye ■ Virtually anything by Marvin Gaye

Table: A sturdy table near the bed can be used to hold drinks, candles, and other items. Make sure that the table is equipped with drawers to provide a discreet place to hold interface safety and enhancement accessories, such as condoms and lubricants.

Storage Area: A built-in storage area, or closet, will provide a space for your clothing and items you want to keep hidden from casual visitors.

Accessories: Stock the closet and/or drawer of the bedside table with your favorite lubes (see chapter 3), foreplay enhancers (see chapters 3 and 6), safety items (see the "Protective Devices" section in this chapter), and sex toys (see chapter 6).

Preparing Your Work Station

It is essential to fully and properly prepare your final sexual work station before entering into the space with a partner. An improperly or incompletely prepared work station can cause frustrating delays and even total sexual-system shutdown.

Sanitize: Remove all visual clutter from the area, including trash, used dishware and glassware, shoes, and articles of clothing. Place them in a storage area (closets or containers) that are hidden from view.

Deodorize: Fumigate the area by opening windows to allow new air to circulate through the premises.

Reodorize: Add a subtle, pleasant odor to the room by burning a scented candle or stick of incense. Alternatively, spritz cologne or perfume in various places around the room.

⚠ *WARNING: Although allergic reactions to incense are uncommon, they do occur. Most allergic reactions to incense occur when it is in liquid form. Typical reactions include skin rash, blueness to the fingers, vomiting, diarrhea, and abdominal pain. If a reaction occurs, it is recommended that you do not induce vomiting. Scented candles can also trigger allergy symptoms, inflame asthma, and induce punishing headaches in some people. Be sensitive to your partner's mood and be prepared to adjust odorization if necessary.*

Temperaturize: Set the work station's thermostat or other climate-control device to a comfortable temperature. The ideal setting is one in which most persons won't feel chilled outside their clothing but will not become over-heated during the rigors of intercourse.

Sanitize: Yes, your final interface work station should provide an environment conducive to sexual arousal, but you should eliminate or hide items that directly refer to sexual activities. Remove posters, books, magazines, and videos depicting sexually desirable models and/or overt sexual acts. Such items may make some people feel inadequate or pressured, thus discouraging sexual interface. Also, be sure to hide photos or video of other current or past sexual partners.

Customize: Beyond the basic components, the general guideline for designing your sexual work station is to make it reflect your personality, "brand," and particular interests. The presentation should enhance the sexual experience, reaffirm your sexual identity, and, ultimately, help your partner to relax.

Protective Devices

Secure any protective devices, such as condoms or cervix caps, and put them in place before beginning intercourse. That way they will be able to perform safely and effectively, right when needed.

Condoms

Condoms (also known as "prophylactics," "rubbers," and "jimmy hats") cover the penis with a thin, synthetic protective layer to prevent the spread of sexually transmitted diseases (STDs) between the genitals during full interface. They also catch and contain sperm emitted from the penis to prevent the spread of viruses as well as unwanted pregnancies.

Be sure to check the expiration date on condom packages and never use a condom that has expired. If you cannot find an expiration date (usually marked as "Exp"), check for the date of manufacture (usually marked as "MFG"). Do not use condoms five years after the manufacture date. Discard condoms containing spermicide two years after the manufacture date.

Condoms come in numerous varieties designed to fit every type of penis, and some may even provide additional stimulation. All types should be stored in a cool, dark, dry place to prevent degradation.

Latex: Strong and durable, latex condoms are highly effective at preventing pregnancy and the spread of disease. However, many people are allergic to latex and can suffer unpleasant side effects as a result of using a latex condom.

Polyurethane: Smoother than latex, polyurethane provides a good alternative to those allergic to latex. It also conducts heat more efficiently and is less likely to cause abrasions. Polyurethane condoms, however, tend to be more expensive and less elastic than latex ones, making them harder to put—and keep—on.

Lambskin: Made from lamb intestines, these condoms are more comfortable than synthetic varieties and prevent the escape of sperm into the vagina just as effectively. But due to their porous molecular structure, they do not provide an effective layer of protection against the spread of STDs.

⚠ *WARNING: Never flush used condoms down a toilet. Because they are made of sturdy, non-water-soluble material, condoms can get trapped in disposal pipes and snare other flushed items, including other used condoms, creating a clog that will be difficult to dislodge.*

Additional Special Features

All condoms commonly available are made of latex, polyurethane, or lambskin, but they often come in numerous specialty brands as well. These include:

Ribbed: Slightly raised bands on the condom can provide additional stimulation for the vagina, though not all people find them stimulating or comfortable.

Studded: Thick, raised bulbs on various spots around the condom can provide additional stimulation for the vagina and clitoris, though some persons find them uncomfortable.

Pleasure Shaped: These specialty condoms fit more loosely and feature enlarged, pouch-like tips. The wider tips allow for more friction because the extra latex stimulates the nerve endings at the tip of the penis. Some also feature a winding, twisting shape that allows for more vigorous action. This design stimulates nerve endings and heightens sensitivity for both women and men.

Desensitizing: Thicker than most varieties, these condoms insulate the penis from intense stimulation during intercourse in an effort to delay orgasm for males worried about premature ejaculation (see chapter 7).

Lubricated: Most condoms come packaged in lubricant to make them easier to apply and more comfortable during intercourse for both partners. However, you still may want to add lubricant after putting it on the penis.

Spermicidal: All lubricants suppress sperm fertility, but the lubricant that these condoms are packaged in contains a substance specifically designed to kill sperm. While offering another layer of protection against pregnancy, the spermicidal substance, however, tends to degrade condoms and increase their likelihood of breaking during intercourse. Some persons are also allergic to spermicide.

Flavored: Designed for oral sex, these condoms add a synthetic fruit or mint flavor to their coating in an effort to make them more pleasant to put in a person's mouth.

⚠ *WARNING: If you plan to use flavored condoms during vaginal sex, make sure they are sugar free. Sugar-flavored condoms can adversely affect the pH in the vagina, which can lead to yeast infections.*

Warming: These condoms contain a warming lubricant that is activated by natural body moisture, so they heat up during sexual intercourse. They are designed to enhance sensual pleasure through the release of gentle, warm sensations for both partners. They also tend to be made of thinner latex, which helps heighten sensation.

Edible: These come in a variety of flavors. They can be rolled on the penis and then eaten off it. Note, however, that edible condoms are for novelty use only. They do not provide any type of protection against pregnancy or sexually transmitted diseases.

Colored: Some condoms come in bright colors, glow in the dark, or provide some other entertaining visual side effect. There are orange condoms for Halloween, green and red condoms for Christmas, even condoms in the colors of various national flags. Many of these "novelty" varieties, however, do not provide a dependable level of protection from pregnancy or STDs. Read the labels and make sure they are as reliable as regular varieties before using one during intercourse.

⚠️ **WARNING:** *Never reuse a condom. Used condoms are much more prone to breakage, placing you and your partner at risk of the spread of STDs and pregnancy.*

Installing a Male Condom

Before installing any condom onto the male penis, be sure to check the expiration date on the packaging to make sure it is not too old to be effective. Condoms past their expiration date are much more likely to tear and burst. Once you have verified that the condom is safe to use, follow these steps for proper installation.

[1] Remove the condom from its packaging. It should be relatively flat, with its base looking like a thick rubber band and its thin, translucent body coiled within the base.

[2] Spread a drop or two of lubricant inside the condom to help it glide more easily onto the penis. (Be careful not to use too much lube or the condom might slip off later.) You can also apply lube to the pubic hair around the base of the penis to keep it from getting snared in the condom.

⚠ **WARNING:** *Use only water- or silicone-based lubricants with condoms. Oil-based lubes can degrade condoms, leading to an increased likelihood of tearing and bursting during intercourse.*

[3] Hold the condom up to let the tip of the body fall below the base. Squeeze the air out of the tip to keep it from bursting during intercourse.

[4] Slide the base of the condom over the glans to the top of the shaft so that the tip of the condom's body fits loosely over the glans.

[5] While pinching the tip with one hand, use the thumb and forefingers of the other hand to roll the base of the condom slowly downward until it reaches the base of the penis, smoothing out any air bubbles along the way.

[6] Check the tip. It should fit loosely over the tip of the glans, with some extra space to catch emitted sperm. Many condoms come with a "reservoir tip," an area at the tip designed for just this purpose. Make sure no air has gotten into the tip, making it swell like a balloon. The air could cause the condom to burst during intercourse. If the tip is full of air, remove the condom and reinstall.

[7] Spread lube over the condom exterior to ease entry into your partner and decrease the risk of tearing.

CONDOM SENSE: Knowing how to properly wear and use a condom car

CONDOMS MAY INCLUDE THE FOLLOWING
SPECIAL FEATURES FOR MAXIMUM
INTERCOURSE PLEASURE:

1. Lubricant
2. Spermicide
3. Assorted flavors

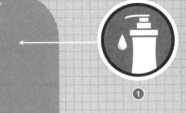

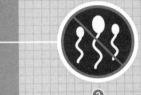

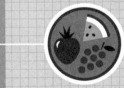

NOTE:
Purchasing condoms can be
intimidating, but knowing you're safe
from disease or unwanted pregnancy
far outweighs any awkward
shopping experience.

make for a safer and more pleasurable sexual interface.

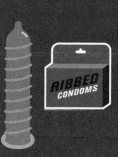 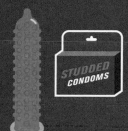 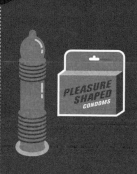

RIBBED CONDOMS

STUDDED CONDOMS

PLEASURE SHAPED CONDOMS

CONDOM TYPES

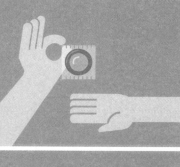 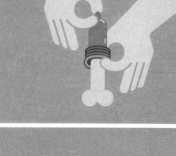

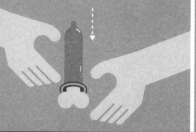 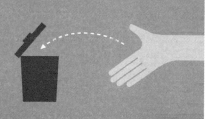

INSTALLATION PROCESS

[8] Occasionally check the condom during intercourse to make sure it has not torn, burst, or fallen off during thrusting.

[9] After ejaculation, remove the penis from the vagina. Grab the base of the condom on either side of your shaft and roll it back up the shaft and over the glans. Enclose the condom in tissue paper and dispose of it in a trash can or other solid-waste receptacle. Try to keep any sperm emitted into the condom from dripping out during removal and disposal. Use this as an opportunity to wipe down the penis as well.

Female Condoms

Condoms also come designed for female genitals. Similar in shape, size, and appearance to their male counterparts, the female condom is slightly longer and wider, with rings at both ends. It provides a protective synthetic liner the full length of the vagina that prevents the passage of sperm or STDs between genitals.

⚠️ **WARNING:** *Never flush used condoms down a toilet. Because they are made of sturdy, non-water-soluble material, condoms can get trapped in disposal pipes and snare other flushed items, including other used condoms, creating a clog that will be difficult to dislodge.*

Installing a Female Condom

As with male condoms, first check the expiration date on the condom's packaging to make sure it is not too old to be effective. Condoms past their expiration date are much more likely to tear and fail.

[1] Remove the condom from its packaging. It should be relatively flat, with two thick rings at either end that look like rubber bands, with a thin, translucent body coiled between.

[2] Spread lubricant over the entrance of and inside the vagina. Also apply to the pubic hair around the vaginal entrance to keep it from getting snared in the condom.

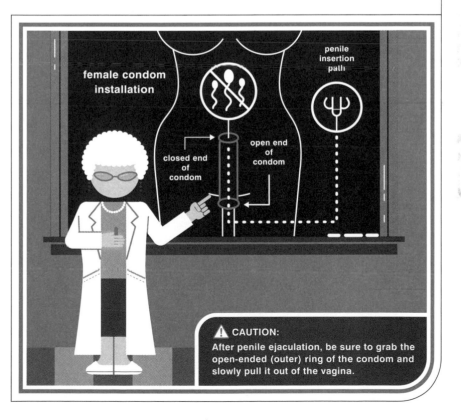

female condom installation

penile insertion path

closed end of condom

open end of condom

⚠ CAUTION:
After penile ejaculation, be sure to grab the open-ended (outer) ring of the condom and slowly pull it out of the vagina.

⚠️ **WARNING:** *Use only water- or silicone-based lubricants with condoms. Oil-based lubes can degrade condoms, leading to an increased likelihood of tearing and bursting during intercourse.*

[**3**] Identify which of the condom rings is slightly smaller in circumference and closed. This side goes toward the back of the vagina.

[**4**] Insert the smaller, closed ring into the vagina, squeezing it if necessary.

[**5**] Use your fingers to push the smaller end into the vagina.

[**6**] Leave the larger, open-ended ring hanging just outside the vaginal entry.

[**7**] Lubricate the penis and insert it into the vagina through the larger, open-ended ring hanging outside the vagina.

[**8**] Allow the penis to slowly push the closed end of the condom up as far as possible into the vagina. Direct the male to use a series of long, slow strokes.

[**9**] After penile ejaculation, grasp the larger, open-ended ring and slowly pull it out of the vagina. Be careful not to allow sperm to drip out of the condom. Wrap the condom in tissue paper and dispose of it in a solid-waste receptacle.

Other Intercourse Protection Devices

In addition to male and female condoms, the market abounds with a variety of devices and products that will ensure some level of protection during sexual interface.

Spermicide: This variety of lubricant includes a substance that kills sperm. It is most effective when used with a condom, diaphragm, cap, sponge, or similar protective device. There are many benefits to spermicide as an intercourse protection method. It is convenient and simple to use, has no effect on a woman's natural hormones, and can be safely used even by women who are breastfeeding. It can be purchased without a prescription at most drugstores and carried in a pocket or purse.

EXPERT TIP: After inserting spermicide, you must wait ten minutes before initializing intercourse. Spermicides typically remain effective for only one hour after insertion. You will need to reinsert spermicide each time you engage in intercourse.

Cervical Cap and Cervical Sponge: These devices are inserted into the back of the vagina to block the movement of sperm from the vagina into the uterus. They prevent pregnancy by keeping the sperm from joining with an egg. Although they offer little protection from STDs, they do provide safeguards against accidental pregnancy. Cervical caps can be inserted up to six hours before sexual activity, providing for uninterrupted sex play. Females should not use a cervical cap if they are allergic to silicone, have poor vaginal muscle tone, or have a history of toxic shock syndrome.

Diaphragm: The diaphragm, or "phragmie," is a shallow, dome-shaped latex cup with a flexible rim. It is inserted into the vagina, blocking access to the uterus and stopping sperm from advancing. To be as effective as possible, the diaphragm should be used with spermicides.

Longer-Lasting and Permanent Protections

Both male and females can limit the chances of accidental pregnancy with various medications and surgical procedures, such as birth control pills and vasectomies.

Birth Control Pills: Oral contraceptives, commonly known as "The Pill," were approved by the U.S. Food and Drug Administration in 1960. Used by 18 million American women each year, the Pill remains one of the most popular forms of pregnancy prevention. There are many different types on the market, and each has its own drug interactions and potential side effects. Consult your physician before deciding on a course of oral contraception.

Vasectomies: This medical procedure prevents the release of sperm when the male ejaculates. It is typically performed by a urologist on an outpatient basis. Every year, some 600,000 men undergo a vasectomy in the United States alone. In a classic vasectomy, testicles and scrotum are cleaned with an antiseptic and possibly shaved. A local anesthetic is injected into the area. The physician then makes one or two small openings in the scrotum. Through the resulting opening, the two vas deferens tubes are cut and then tied, stitched, or sealed. The vas deferens is then put back inside the scrotum and the skin is closed with stitches that eventually dissolve. In recent years, a less invasive form of the procedure called a no-scalpel vasectomy has grown in popularity. Consult your physician before undergoing this procedure.

Basic Intercourse Mechanics

Although performed in a multitude of positions and tempos, the basic mechanics of intercourse involve the insertion of a fully activated penis into a fully activated vagina. Both partners then manipulate their body positions and various muscles to move the penis up and down the vagina, with the pace and depth of the thrusting, as well as its duration, dependent upon the preferences and capabilities of the participating parties. Here are a few pointers.

[1] Establish and maintain eye contact during the early stages of intercourse. This will help you gauge your partner's reactions and need for adjustments. Sustained eye contact can also heighten erotic software activation and intensify physical and emotional pleasure.

[2] Do not rush through the early stages of intercourse. Slowly work the penis into the vagina, making sure it is lubricated and wide enough to accommodate it. Once the penis is fully inserted into the vagina, pause to allow the vagina to further expand, lubricate, and accustom itself to the penis. Do not begin moving the penis up and down the vaginal canal until the female signals that she is fully prepared to proceed. Then begin with gentle, shallow thrusting, increasing the pace and depth only after the female indicates she is ready. This approach will minimize the chances of discomfort and injury and optimize the potential for pleasure and intimacy.

[3] If you or your partner experiences emotional or physical discomfort, stop. Continuing could lead to serious injury and a lengthy sexual-system shutdown. Take a break and assess. Discuss the problems you are encountering with your partner. Then make adjustments to eliminate discomfort before resuming, or return to foreplay mode.

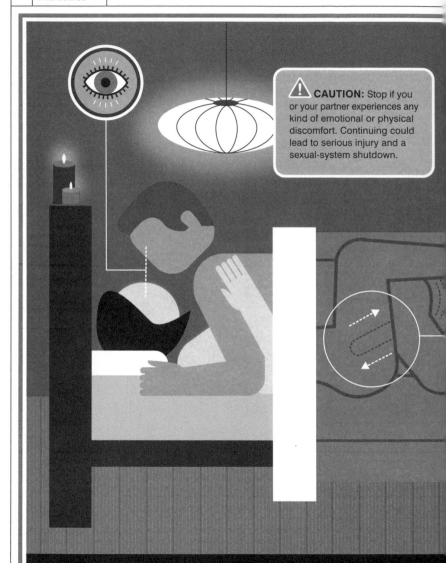

CAUTION: Stop if you or your partner experiences any kind of emotional or physical discomfort. Continuing could lead to serious injury and a sexual-system shutdown.

BASIC SEXUAL TRAINING: When engaging in sexual interface wit

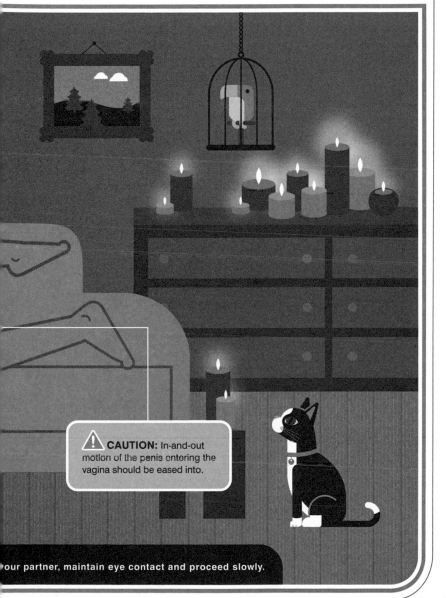

CAUTION: In-and-out motion of the penis entering the vagina should be eased into.

our partner, maintain eye contact and proceed slowly.

INTERCOURSE POSITIONS

Core Intercourse Positions

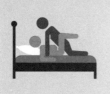

MISSIONARY:
Female lies on her back and spreads her legs while lifting her buttocks and genitals slightly. The male moves between her legs and inserts his penis into her vagina. Because of its face-to-face intimacy and opportunity to maintain constant mouth contact and communication, the Missionary serves as a good starting position for many couples.

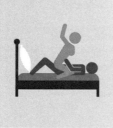

COWGIRL:
Male lies on his back. Female straddles his genitals and lowers her vagina onto his penis. This position can be difficult to master and may prove too acrobatic for some, but it does provide the female more control, along with a less strenuous option for the male. It also allows the male free use of his hands to manually stimulate her breasts, buttocks, and other erotically charged body parts.

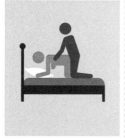

CANINE:
Commonly known as "doggy style" or just "doggy." Female kneels on all fours and raises her buttocks slightly to expose her genitals to the rear; male crouches behind her and enters her vagina from behind. This position allows for deeper thrusting and the stimulation of breasts, buttocks, etc.

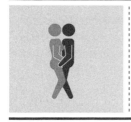

STANDING:

Male and female stand facing each other, with male inserting his penis from below as female raises one leg to ease entry. Difficult to engineer, this position does offer face-to-face intimacy and the chance to practice in unusual places without a bed or comfortable reclining option.

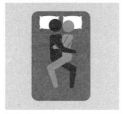

SIDE BY SIDE:

Male and female lie on a bed on their sides facing each other; she lifts one leg to ease entry. This position offers the intimacy of Missionary with a greater sense of equality between partners, along with a gentler pace and new stimulation possibilities.

Test these positions, taking the time to learn each with your partner. Through slight adjustments, you can customize each to accommodate the particular preferences and needs of both persons. All also feature numerous variations that can provide variety and additional stimulation.

Missionary Variations

Basic intercourse activities can prove extremely rewarding for both participants. Yet, trying out advanced techniques will add variety to your sex life and may even lead to the discovery of positions and techniques that provide even greater pleasure.

These simple adjustments may allow for increased pleasure during intercourse in the Missionary position.

⚠ *WARNING: Due to changes in thrusting angles, many of these positions increase the likelihood of the penis slipping out of the vagina during intercourse. If this happens and you do not stop before the next thrust, the penis could get bent between your bodies, resulting in serious injury. Proceed more slowly and cautiously when performing intercourse in these variations, particularly when first trying one out.*

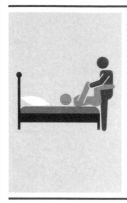

MAN UP:

The man stands at the edge of the bed while the female lies with her back on the bed, positioning her genitals as close to the edge of the bed as possible. The man enters from above and remains standing while thrusting downward. This position can provide more stimulation for the penis and the vagina. Also, by letting the man's leg muscles take over the majority of the thrusting movement, it allows for more vigorous penetration and provides a good alternative for men whose stomach and buttocks muscles are tiring from thrusting in the regular Missionary position.

EXPERT TIP: *Vigorous thrusting is unnecessary for intense stimulation in many positions, particularly those that allow for deeper penetration. After the penis has been inserted into the vaginal canal, adjust postures so that parts of the male genitals push against the G-spot and/or clitoris. Then proceed with short, quick thrusts that keep the penis in continual contact with the G-spot and/or clitoris. This method offers a good break from the vigorous exertion of full thrusting and can actually be more stimulating for both participants.*

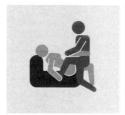

LEGS ENTWINED:

After insertion, the male moves one leg to the outside of the female's leg on the same side while keeping his other leg between her legs. By adjusting the thrusting angle, this position offers a different variety of stimulation for both sets of genitals.

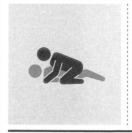

LEGS SWITCH:

After inserting his penis into the vagina, the male lifts his legs, one at a time, and places them on the outside of the legs of the female as she moves her legs together. While it may take a little time to get used to the shallower, curved thrusting motion required by this position, it does provide additional stimulation for the female's clitoris.

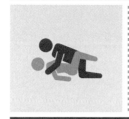

LEGS RAISED AND BENT:
The female lifts her legs, bends them at the knees and places them along the sides of his chest. This position provides greater stimulation of the G-spot and increased thrusting power for the male.

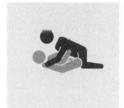

LEGS RAISED AND BENT, FEET ON CHEST:
The female raises her legs, bends her knees, and places her feet on the chest and/or shoulders of the male. This position offers more control of thrusting depth and tempo for the female.

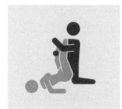

LEGS RAISED, OVER TO ONE SIDE:
The female raises her legs straight up after insertion, then moves them both onto either the left or right shoulder of the male.

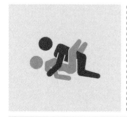

LEGS WRAPPED:
The female wraps her legs around the back of the male and joins her ankles, providing a different penetration angle and increased genital stimulation.

EXPERT TIP: *A simple yet highly effective variation on the Missionary position: Place a pillow under the female's buttocks. Doing so doesn't require additional stretching by the female, and the pillow will push her genitals upward and back, creating a new angle that allows for deeper penetration and greater G-spot stimulation.*

Advanced Missionary Variations

These variations tend to require more dexterity, flexibility, and practice. Proceed with caution when trying them for the first time, and don't hesitate to call off the experiment if it's causing either person discomfort.

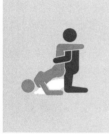

LEGS RAISED AND DRAPED:
After entry, the female raises her legs, bending them at the knees, and then drapes them over the shoulders of the male. This position does require a fair amount of flexibility and caution, but the payoff can be huge: It allows for deeper penetration and more stimulation of the G-spot. By using her legs, the female can also finesse the angle of penetration for maximum stimulation.

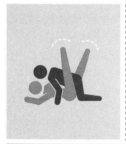

V LEGS:
The female raises her legs straight up and slightly to the sides to form a V and pistons them next to the male's body, then a few inches away, to help propel his thrusts.

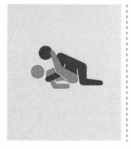

LEGS OVERHEAD:
After insertion, the female raises her legs and bends them straight back so that the knees touch her own shoulders and feet extend over her head.

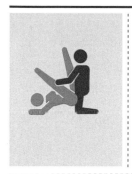

SPREAD-EAGLED:

After insertion, the female extends her legs as wide as possible to each side, as though performing "the splits."

⚠ **WARNING:** *Because the female's groin muscles are stretched so far in the Spread-Eagled position, the male needs to thrust with extreme caution to avoid injuring her.*

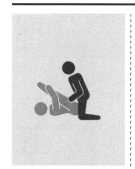

YOGA POSE:

Assume the position described in Legs Overhead. Next, the female moves her arms to the inside and up and around her upper leg to grab her own ankles. This move requires extreme flexibility on the part of the female.

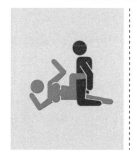

CAMEL RIDE:

The female lies on her side with her top leg forward. The man kneels astride the woman's lower leg, thus gaining access to the vagina. This is good for pregnant or overweight partners.

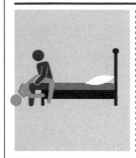

WATERFALL:
After basic Missionary penetration, the female leans back, letting her upper body spill over the side of the bed as the male holds her hips. After she positions her head and shoulders in a stable and comfortable position on the floor, he begins thrusting.

⚠ **WARNING:** *The male should refrain from thrusting too hard in the Waterfall position to prevent injuring the female's neck. Place pillows beneath her head, neck, and shoulders for safety and comfort.*

Female on Top (Cowgirl) Variations

Woman-on-top positions provide an effective change of pace. These adjustments can make sexual intercourse even more exciting and pleasurable.

⚠ **WARNING:** *When first trying these positions, pay careful attention to additional stress placed on both persons' backs, knees, buttocks, neck, and leg muscles. Proceed slowly to avoid causing hardware malfunction.*

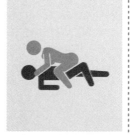

LYING COWGIRL:
Essentially, the Missionary position in reverse, with the female lying atop the male. Note that instead of thrusting, you can achieve intense stimulation through simple bouncing. After deep insertion in a Cowgirl position, both partners quickly move up and down, just an inch or two, as their groins bounce off each other. This motion provides constant and intense stimulation of both partners' genitals.

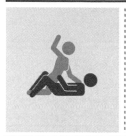

LEGS REVERSED:

The male puts his legs to the outside of the female's while she moves her legs together. This can greatly increase the stimulation on the clitoris.

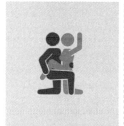

BENDED KNEE:

Both partners kneel facing each other. The female raises her left leg and places it over the top of his right thigh while he reaches his left arm around her lower back for support. After penis insertion, both partners move slowly back and forth toward each other, with her left leg lifting and lowering slightly to help propel the thrusts.

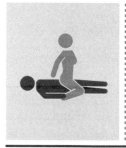

COWGIRL CANINE:

The female turns her back to the male, then slowly lowers her vagina onto his penis. Although it prevents face-to-face intimacy, this posture does afford him a prime view of her buttocks and allows the male to use his hands to reach around to stimulate her clitoris as well as her breasts. He can also lie back while she leans forward on her hands to stimulate different parts of her genitals.

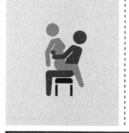

THE ARCH:

The male sits on a stool or chair with his feet planted firmly on either side. The female lowers her vagina onto his penis. Both partners enjoy more thrusting power and control, and having his feet on the ground helps limit lower-back stress. By slightly adjusting the pelvis, both partners can easily create more stimulating penetration angles.

Advanced Female on Top (Cowgirl) Variations

RECLINED:
After assuming basic Cowgirl position, the female leans back, resting her hands on the bed, bends her knees, and rests her feet to either side of his buttocks. The position requires both parties to concentrate so they can synchronize the thrusts, which take on a more curved motion. For a variation on this variation, she can put her legs over his shoulders or lean forward and rest her hands on his shoulders.

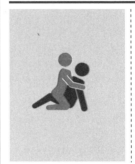

MILKING:
A woman with strong vaginal muscles can assume the Cowgirl position and then tighten and loosen her vagina around the penis without moving the rest of her body. This provides the female with a great sense of control and the male with an opportunity to rest while still receiving an intense and unique form of stimulation.

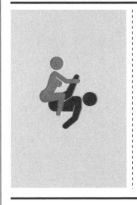

LEANING:
After insertion, the male raises his knees to his chest while the female rises into a squatting position and leans on the back of his legs and buttocks, steadying herself by placing her hands on his ankles. The position can be difficult to get into and places a lot of strain on both partners' upper legs and lower backs. But it affords the female more control than in almost any other position, allowing her to dictate the depth and tempo of thrusting. This position can also be done in a Canine posture with her buttocks facing him.

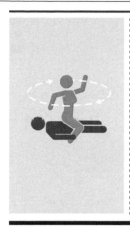

SPINNING:

The female lowers onto his penis in the basic Cowgirl position, then, steadying herself, turns her body slowly, a quarter-turn to the right, so that her right hip faces his chest. After a period of gentle thrusting, she performs another quarter-turn so that her buttocks is facing his chin. Then, after some thrusting, she turns again so that her left hip faces his chest. After more thrusting, she turns once more so that she is back in basic Cowgirl. This sequence can prove challenging and requires concentration and cooperation to avoid injury. But it offers a variety of new stimulations as the penis pushes against different parts of the vagina.

Standing Variations

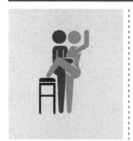

LEG UP AND TO SIDE:

The female places one leg out to the side, resting it on a chair or other item. This posture allows for easier penetration and adjustment during thrusting, to increase stimulation.

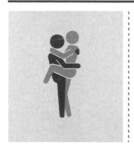

LEG UP AND AROUND MALE:

The female lifts one leg and wraps it around the male's buttocks or thighs. This position gives her greater control of the thrusting tempo, depth, and angle.

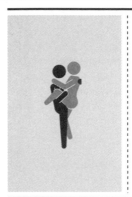

LEG UP AND HELD:
The female lifts one leg, allowing him to cradle it with his arm on the same side.

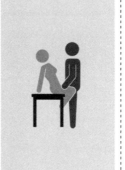

STANDING TO SEATED:
The female sits or reclines on a desktop, table, or other sturdy object, and he stands in front of her and enters. This position can provide intense stimulation for both and with less effort. It can also be employed in a variety of locations outside the bedroom.

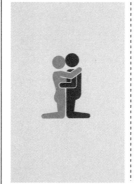

KNEELING:
Both partners kneel facing each other. The male then enters the female. This position affords greater intimacy, gentler thrusting, and easier adjustment of penetration angles than in most other standing positions.

Advanced Standing Variations

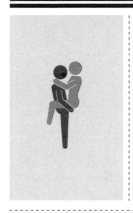

HOLDING:
The male places his hands on her buttocks or back of her thighs and lifts, holding her in the air as thrusting continues. This move can provide intense stimulation but requires great strength from him.

⚠ **EXPERT TIP:** *To ease some of the stress on the male's legs, arms, and back during the Holding position, you can adjust your bodies into the "Harvey Wallbanger" posture. The woman leans back against a wall or other sturdy object to ease some of the weight off the male. This position can offer the opportunity for intense thrusting. Just make sure the wall or supporting apparatus does not grate against her skin.*

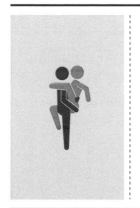

LEG UP AND OVER SHOULDER:
The female lifts one leg and places it over the male's corresponding shoulder just prior to or after penetration. This posture requires that she be extremely flexible and not prone to leg cramps.

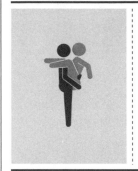

BOTH LEGS OVER SHOULDERS:
The female raises one leg over his shoulder, and he cradles her other leg and helps her raise it over his other shoulder. Exciting for some persons, this position requires extreme flexibility and can create difficulties in achieving and maintaining a good thrusting angle. It may also be difficult to keep the penis from falling out of the vagina.

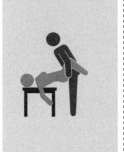

FALL BACK:
After achieving penetration and going into Holding position, the male slowly lowers the upper half of the female's body to the ground, then thrusts downward. Some couples find this position highly stimulating, but be sure the upper half of the female's body is resting in a comfortable position and on a secure surface.

Canine Variations

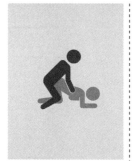

FLATTENED CANINE:
After penetration in Basic Canine, she leans downward onto her forearms while he puts first one knee, then the other, on each side of her buttocks while also lowering his hips. May be uncomfortable for some, but highly stimulating for others.

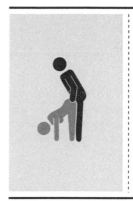

STANDING CANINE:
Both partners stand, with his groin against her buttocks. Then the female bends over from the waist, and he enters her from behind. She can place her hands against a wall, desk, or the floor for stability.

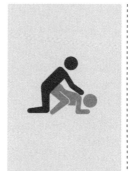

SQUATTING CANINE:
The female squats (instead of leans) in front of the male as he kneels behind her and enters. The position affords more control for her, but she will need strong legs to sustain it for long periods.

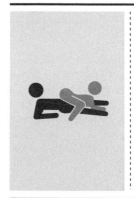

REVERSE COWGIRL:
The male lies on his back and the female places her knees on either side of his hips with her buttocks toward his face, then lowers her vagina onto his penis and bends her knees under her. The position affords her more control and gives him a prime view of her buttocks.

Advanced Canine Variations

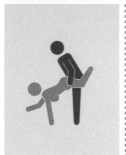

WHEELBARROWING:
The female rests her forearms on the floor and the male grabs her thighs to raise her legs and enter her from behind. For a further twist, she can move across the floor by walking on her hands as he thrusts from behind. Also known as "The Hoover Maneuver."

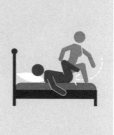

LAWN CHAIR:
The male lies with his back on the bed and knees raised halfway to his chest. The female turns her back to him and lowers her vagina onto his penis and the back of his thighs, as though sitting onto a low lawn chair. The position affords her great control and frees her hands to stimulate his scrotum or slap his buttocks.

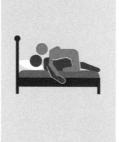

LEAN BACK:
The male lies with his back on the bed; she stands with her back to him and lowers her vagina onto his penis with her knees bent and placed on either side of his hips. The female then leans all the way back so that her back touches his chest and her knees remain bent under her. This position can be difficult to get into, but it allows the male to manually stimulate the female's breasts and clitoris during thrusting.

Side-by-Side Variations

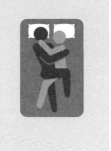

LEG WRAP:
After penetration in the basic side-by-side position, the male wraps his legs around her waist. This allows for deeper thrusting and extra protection against the penis falling out during intercourse. During a long intercourse session, you may have to roll onto the other side to avoid having his leg "fall asleep" beneath her.

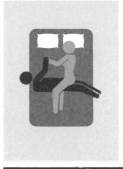

LOWERING DOWN:
After penetration in the basic Side-by-Side posture, the male rotates his body downward so that it approaches a 90-degree angle to the female's, instead of being parallel. Be careful that the penis does not slip out of the vagina during repositioning and keep thrusts shallow.

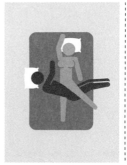

SCISSORING:
The female lies on her side and lifts one leg while the male lies on his side and gets between her legs at a 90-degree angle from her, as if forming a cross, and enters.

Intercourse and Menstruation

During the time in life between maturation and menopause, females experience a period of menstruation a few days every month, during which the lining of the uterus sheds and blood exits via the vaginal opening. Known commonly as a "period," this phenomenon can also lead to bloating, vaginal cramping, and mood swings. Other commonly used appellations for menstruation include "the monthlies" and "visits from Aunt Flo."

It is best not to attempt intercourse during menstruation, for it can cause great discomfort and a messy discharge. The pieces of the uterine lining can also rub against the vagina during thrusting, leading to injury and long-term discomfort. Menstrual blood can also act as a highly efficient conduit for many sexually transmitted diseases, such as HIV.

If you want to try intercourse during menstruation, be sure to use a condom and put a towel or other protective device beneath you to soak up discharge and to prevent it from staining surfaces. Also, avoid Cowgirl positions to lessen excessive discharge. Proceed very slowly to protect against injury to the vagina. Or just try an alternative to intercourse, such as manual stimulation.

Anal Intercourse

Difficult to master and, for many, difficult to even begin, the act of plugging the penis into the anus can provide intense and unique stimulation for both partners. It may serve as an alternative during female menstruation. Using a strap-on synthetic penis (commonly known as a "strapadictomy"), females and males can also switch positions and get a sense of how the other partner feels during regular intercourse.

⚠ *WARNING: If the person being penetrated complains of pain during anal sex, stop immediately. Though a little discomfort is natural in the early stages of the activity, pain can indicate tearing of the anus or other injury.*

Hygiene

Because the main function of the anus is to dispense fecal waste, it can be a prime source of germs and unpleasant odors. Make sure to empty the bowels and bathe prior to attempting anal sex, scrubbing the anus with soap.

It is equally important to clean up after anal sex. The penis should be thoroughly washed with warm soap and water, and then washed again. The anus that was penetrated also needs to be scrubbed clean. Anal toys should be used with condoms or sterilized after each use.

💡 *EXPERT TIP: In addition to aiding hygiene, a long, hot bath before anal sex helps relax the rectal muscles and ease penetration and thrusting.*

Anal Foreplay

Anal sex requires extra lubrication to ease entry into and up the anal canal. Apply liberal amounts of lubricant to both the penis and the anal opening.

To prepare the anus for penetration by an actual or synthetic penis, first use a well-lubricated finger and ease it into the anus. The sphincter, a tight band of muscle around the anus, will tighten around your finger. Let it slowly relax by gently swirling your finger around the anus. Work your finger gently up and down the anal canal.

EXPERT TIP: Some people enjoy having a finger inserted into their anus during oral sex or intercourse. Loosening the sphincter and stimulating the prostate can actually lead to more prolonged and intense orgasms for males. The prostate, or P-Spot, is a walnut-sized and similarly shaped gland located just inside the front wall of the rectal canal, a few inches from the anal opening. It can be stimulated with a penis or by inserting a finger into the anal canal and rubbing its inside wall. Not all persons enjoy this activity, so be sure to discuss it before and during the procedure.

Penetration

Approach the tip of the penis to the anus and slowly ease it inside. The sphincter will likely tighten around the penis and even attempt to expel it. Take your time and let the sphincter relax before penetrating any further.

As the sphincter relaxes, ease the penis farther up the anal canal. Gently move it up and down the canal. Pay close attention to your partner's responses to gauge how quickly and deeply you should thrust.

Instead of thrusting, you can just vibrate your buttocks, pelvis, and penis to create additional stimulation. This action may help relax the sphincter or offer a pleasurable alternative to thrusting.

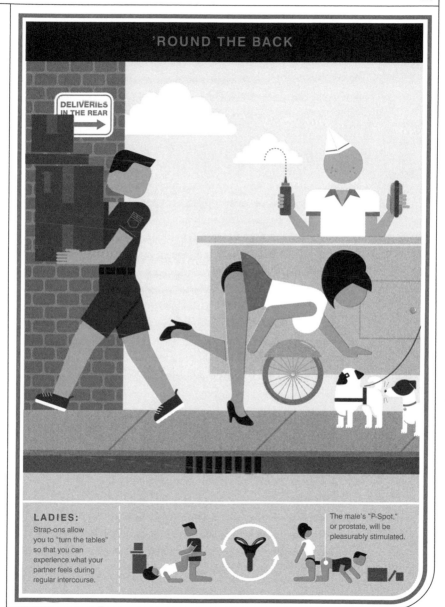

'ROUND THE BACK

DELIVERIES
IN THE REAR

LADIES:
Strap-ons allow
you to "turn the tables"
so that you can
experience what your
partner feels during
regular intercourse.

The male's "P-Spot,"
or prostate, will be
pleasurably stimulated.

⚠️ **EXPERT TIP:** *Though it seems counterintuitive, flexing the buttocks cheeks together just prior to penetration can actually ease anal entry and allow for quick, deep penetration.*

Positions

Use the basic positions and their variations (excluding the Female on Top postures). However, because the angle of penetration is significantly different during anal sex, you will need to slightly adjust your posture. It is also important that the recipient can exert some control over thrusting tempo and intensity. Anal sex can be quite uncomfortable, especially during the early stages. Controlling the process will help the receiver relax, ease into the activity, and gain greater enjoyment.

⚠️ **WARNING:** *Anal sex is even riskier than vaginal intercourse, especially for the recipient. Condoms offer protection from HIV and other sexually transmitted diseases, but they stand a greater chance of tearing during anal sex. Use stronger condoms, proper technique, and plenty of lubricant to avoid condom failure during anal intercourse.*

Orgasm

Whether intended for pleasure or for facilitating impregnation, most sexual encounters seek orgasm as an end result. The phenomenon usually occurs after intense genital stimulation and involves a relatively brief interlude of great pleasure, pelvic muscle contraction, and a feeling of general euphoria and release. The process is roughly similar for male and females alike, but it involves different hardware, along with some variations in cause, effect, and results.

Male Orgasm

Male climax is associated and usually concurrent with ejaculation, the expulsion of fluid through the urothral opening on the glans. However, the two actually represent separate phenomena. Males can ejaculate without orgasm, and they can orgasm without ejaculation.

Male orgasm specifically involves a series of contractions of pelvic muscles around the genitals and anus. The contractions, which last from a few seconds to half a minute, start at about one-second intervals, then slow as they continue. (Duration of orgasmic contractions tends to diminish with age, as does the amount of semen ejaculated during orgasm.) Most males will also experience changes in body temperature, with flushing in certain parts of their body, as well as changes in their breathing and heart rates.

During orgasmic contractions, seminal fluid produced in the testicles and prostate is usually pushed up through the penis and ejaculated via the urethral opening on the glans; because of the force of the orgasmic muscle contractions, it generally exits in spurts. The fluid contains numerous materials, including millions of sperm, just one of which can fertilize an egg in the female's uterus. Sperm can remain viable outside the male body for up to several days.

Post-Orgasm for Males

Following orgasm, most males experience a de-erection of the penis plus general relaxation and even fatigue. These effects are due to the release into the brain of endorphins—so-called happy hormones—that reduce stress and induce a feeling of calmness. As a result, many post-climax males will fall asleep or feel intensely hungry.

Because it takes most males a long time to reactivate their genitals to achieve another orgasm, and many become fatigued or disinterested after

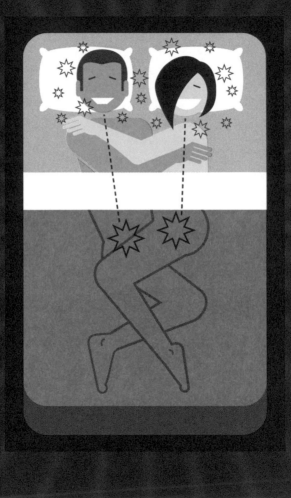

the first orgasm, the length of time required for them to climax plays a crucial role in the sexual encounter. Males who orgasm before their partners, and then discontinue the session, can engender anger and frustration instead of joy and satisfaction in their partners. Both parties should consult with each other beforehand about the male's past experiences so that you can gauge the approximate amount of time he will require to climax. Adjust your approach and expectations accordingly.

EXPERT TIP: Simultaneous orgasm ranks as one of the most heralded and sought-after goals for couples attempting sexual interface. Beware: Consciously attempting to coordinate orgasms can leave both partners frustrated and may prohibit the achievement of individual orgasm. Couples are usually better advised to concentrate on taking care of one person's orgasm, and then the other's, leaving simultaneous orgasms to happen when (and if) they will.

Female Orgasm

Though some females are capable of ejaculating fluid through their urethra during orgasms (see "Female Ejaculation" later in this chapter), sexual climax for most occurs internally. In addition, most females are capable of two different types of orgasm: clitoral and vaginal, or G-spot. Most females find that G-spot orgasms tend to be deeper and more relaxing, while clitoral climaxes are quicker and more intense.

Both types of female orgasm involve the contraction of muscles around the genitals. The contractions, which last from a few seconds to almost a minute, start at about one-second intervals, then slow as they continue. Like males, most females will experience changes in body temperature, with flushing in certain parts of their hardware, along with changes in breathing and heart rates.

Most female orgasms occur after prolonged and direct manipulation of the genitals; clitoral orgasms resulting from stimulation of the clitoris, and G-spot orgasms resulting from stimulation of the G-spot. Oral, manual, or intergenital stimulation of the clitoris and G-spot usually builds through repetition and slight variation of manipulative exercises until they inspire orgasm. Foreplay has a crucial role in preparing the female genitals for direct stimulation and orgasm, as well as in activating the psychological software necessary for orgasm.

Post-Orgasm for Females

Postorgasmic behavior varies among females. Some grow more aroused and want to continue being genitally stimulated to achieve additional orgasms; others become fatigued or sore and want to rest or cease sexual activities.

Some females orgasm very quickly after the initiation of genital manipulation. Others require up to an hour. Many females find it difficult or even impossible to orgasm no matter how long they are stimulated (see "Addressing Sexual Malfunctions," page 195). The amount of time it takes to achieve orgasm may also depend on the female's current physical and emotional state.

Many females can orgasm multiple times during a relatively brief period without becoming fatigued. Others can achieve only one per interface session, and sometimes not even that. Consult with your partner about her orgasmic frequency tendencies, and adjust your approach and expectations accordingly.

Female Ejaculation

Some females expel a clear fluid through their urethral opening during G-spot orgasm. The exact nature and origin of the liquid remains uncertain, though most of it seems to come from near the Skene's gland and resemble female urine. Some find this expulsion erotic, but others do not, particularly if they are in the process of orally servicing the genitals of the ejaculator. If you frequently ejaculate, discuss it with your partner before oral manipulation of your genitals.

Enhancing Orgasms

Orgasms mark the height of physical and emotional pleasure for most people. You can increase the intensity of your orgasmic experience by employing these techniques.

Multiple Stimulation: Many persons forget about stimulation efforts of the breasts and other hardware once they have moved on to genital stimulation. However, returning to this activity as you continue to stimulate the genitals can lead to greater orgasm intensity. Just use a free hand or your mouth to stimulate the nipples, neck, lips, or other erogenous zones.

Teasing: Although difficult to master, teasing can greatly increase both the physical and psychological intensity and duration of orgasm. Stimulate yourself or your partner to the brink of orgasm, then pause in your efforts until the urge to orgasm recedes. Restart until the brink of orgasm is reached again, then pause again. Repeat several times, increasing the rate of stimulation as orgasm approaches and then finally allow it to occur. If you are performing this technique on a partner, closely audit the changes in physical state as orgasm approaches. Gauging the rate of breathing, vocalizations, posture, and muscle responses will help you spot an impend-ing orgasm and stop stimulation efforts before it's too late.

⚠️ **WARNING:** *Drugs that promise to increase the intensity of orgasms should be avoided. They can be dangerous, and most actually distract, delay, or even prevent climax. The orgasm represents the ultimate high and does not need synthetic chemical compounds to improve it. Similarly, folk remedies, such as drinking pickle juice, have not been proved to delay or intensify orgasm or stave off loss of erection in males.*

Massage: A full-body massage prior to genital manipulation can help the body relax and increase blood flow. Concentrate on the muscles around the groin, buttocks, neck, and head. Reducing stress and increasing blood flow to the genitals and brain can lead to easier and more pleasurable orgasms.

Opening Posture: Many people close up their bodies during genital stimu-lation, crossing their arms over their chests, pushing their legs together and grimacing with their facial muscles. Relax your face by opening your mouth. Spread-eagle during genital stimulation. Such postures will help calm your muscles and mind, increase blood flow, and give yourself over to an orgasm.

Vibrators: A vibrating sex toy applied to the genitals or other erogenous zones during, or as a substitute for, oral, manual, or intergenital stimulation can greatly increase pleasure and orgasm intensity. "Vibes," as they are commonly known, can actually be overwhelming for some persons and body parts, so progress slowly to find the optimal level of stimulation.

Increased Vocalization: Due to embarrassment or privacy issues, many peo-ple try to stifle the noises they make leading up to and during orgasm. Allow yourself and/or your partner to increase the volume, frequency, and range of vocabulary of vocalization. This release can lead to greater awareness, increased feedback to your partner, and effective adjustment of stimulation efforts, not to mention a quicker and more intense orgasm. Just make sure you apply this technique in a private place where no one can hear you so that you can vocalize as loudly and as often as you like.

Health Benefits of Orgasm

If you have problems with your heart, blood flow, or general health, consult with a doctor to make sure your body can handle sexual climax. For those who can, orgasm offers several mental and physical health benefits. Because the heart races leading up to and during sexual climax, orgasm provides a good cardio workout. It also releases tension, helping ease muscle strain, cramps, and emotional stress.

In addition, orgasm provides pain relief, as the body floods with endorphins, a highly effective natural painkiller. Regular sex and orgasm can also help stave off the effects of aging, according to some researchers.

Orgasm is not a substitute for exercise, psychological counseling, lifestyle changes to help reduce stress, or medical attention for a problem causing you physical discomfort. But it can provide effective, temporary relief and benefits that you can build on.

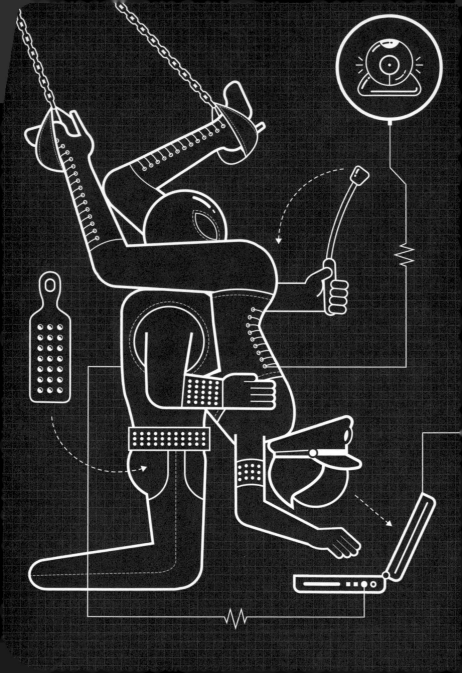

Chapter 5

Advanced Sexual Interface

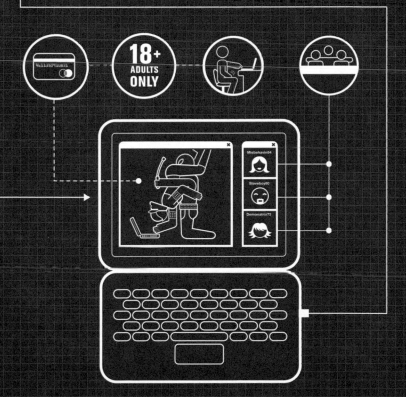

So far, we have discussed the most conventional techniques of achieving orgasm—and for many people, these techniques offer enough variety for a lifetime of sexual fulfillment.

But the world offers an infinite number of ways to enhance your sex life. The Internet has introduced countless new opportunities for people with like-minded interests to meet and engage with partners online. Kinks and fetishes allow people to obtain sexual gratification from ordinary household objects. And of course pornography has never been more accessible or affordable. In fact, you probably have the necessary technology to create your own.

Anyone in search of "something different" can treat this list as a good place to start.

⚠ *WARNING: Depending on your experience, the activities described below may seem unconventional and even immoral—but they are certainly not illegal. If you can pursue your desires with the help of a consenting adult(s) (without violating the rights of any other living creature), you're on safe ground. But if you believe that you and/or your partner may be flirting with the boundaries of unlawful or unhealthy alternative activities, we urge you to seek professional help immediately.*

Common Alternatives

Remote Sex: Using technological devices, such as telephones or computers, to exchange sexual messages with a partner while you occupy two different spaces, along with one or both partners usually engaging in self-stimulation. Phone sex, "cybersex" conducted in online chat rooms or via instant messaging system, and "cam-to-cam" (or "C2C") encounters are all common acts of remote sex.

⚠ **WARNING:** *Cybersex can be a great way to explore fantasies and avoid unwanted emotional entanglements. But anonymity also has its pitfalls. Be very careful with whom you enter into a cybersex relationship. If at all possible, demand a recent photograph and pay close attention to the content of the messages you receive. You can usually determine your partner's age by his or her language. Never engage in cybersex communication with anyone you suspect may not be of legal age. Also, be sure to keep your personal information private. Never give out your home phone number until you have established a level of comfort with your partner.*

Threesomes and Group Sex: Engaging in sexual activities simultaneously with more than one partner. A three-way sexual encounter is commonly referred to as a "ménage à trois," whereas group sex sessions are known as "orgies." (See page 169 for more information.)

Body Part Fetishism: Focusing the majority of attention during sexual interface on a body part other than the genitals. Common body part fetishes include the feet, breasts, legs, and buttocks, but can include anything from the ears to the eyebrows. Many foot fetishists also become fixated with footwear and foot decoration. Their interest in feet may come with an attendant fascination with shoes, stockings, nail polish, foot binding, pedicures, and even foot odor.

Fashion Play: Engaging in sexual activities with someone dressed in a costume, particular style of clothing, a particular clothing item, or clothing made from a particular material such as latex or leather. Some common fashion fetishes include leather, cowboy boots, firefighter uniforms, stockings, bowler hats, high heels, cycling shorts, and neckties.

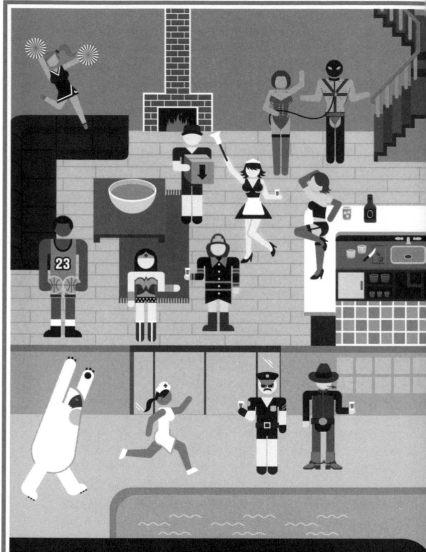

FASHION PLAY: Costumes can add another level of excitement to a sexual situation.

157

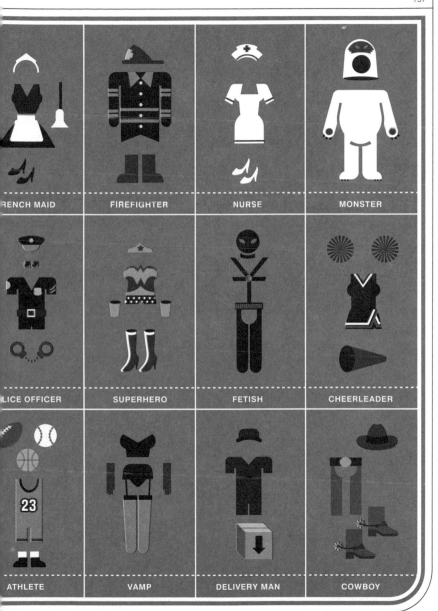

FRENCH MAID

FIREFIGHTER

NURSE

MONSTER

POLICE OFFICER

SUPERHERO

FETISH

CHEERLEADER

ATHLETE

VAMP

DELIVERY MAN

COWBOY

Food Play: Incorporating food or beverages into sexual activities, such as licking whipped cream off a lover's nipple. Specific substrata of food play involve sex with sausages (or other phallus-shaped meats), attempts to penetrate foods that mimic the vagina or anus (such as pies and fruits), and so-called wakame sake, a sexual act that entails drinking rice wine off a woman's mons pubis. Food play has been depicted repeatedly in popular culture, most memorably in the novel *Portnoy's Complaint* and the popular film *American Pie*.

Swinging: Openly exchanging partners with another couple or group of couples. The swinging scene is most closely associated with the 1970s and has been depicted in numerous books, feature films, and television shows. These include the acclaimed novels *The Ice Storm* by Rick Moody and *The 158-Pound Marriage* by John Irving; the film *Bob & Carol & Ted & Alice*; and the TV series *Swingtown* and *Six Feet Under*. *The Ice Storm* and its ensuing film adaptation helped popularize the notion of "key parties" at which husbands would deposit their keys into a large bowl at the start of the party and then have their wives pull the keys out of the bowl and have sex with whomever's keys they ended up with.

Talking Dirty: Exchanging obscene comments about each other and what you want to do to each other before, during, or after sex. Dirty talk may include the sharing of fantasies, including transgressive fantasies involving rape or group sex, that may not reflect actual sexual aspirations and preferences.

Tantric: Practicing ancient sexual exercises to gain deeper satisfaction and more profound spiritual connection with your interface partner. Tantric sex was popularized in recent years by pop star Sting, who claimed in an interview that he used tantric techniques to have uninterrupted sex for six hours.

Exhibitionism: The exposure of breasts, buttocks, or genitals in public settings (or in private settings where passing bystanders might witness them, such as the window of an apartment building). Many people practice this activity simply by dressing in provocative clothing. Others take the activity one step further by exposing their genitals, buttocks, or breasts and by engaging in public sex acts; note that both variations are illegal throughout most of the United States.

Voyeurism: Watching others engage in sexual or nonsexual activities. Here again, many people practice this activity on a daily basis simply by walking around a neighborhood on their lunch hour. If you observe a person in his/her private space without obtaining express permission, you are breaking the law.

B&D (Bondage and Discipline): Restraining of one partner by the other and/or punishment for bad behavior through spanking or other disciplinary actions. Often lumped together with sadism and masochism under the rubric BDSM.

D&S (Dominance and Submission): Surrendering control, with one partner agreeing to do whatever the other demands. Often coupled with B&D.

S&M (Sadism and Masochism): Gaining sexual pleasure by inflicting pain on a partner (sadism) or enduring pain from a partner (masochism). Often coupled with B&D and/or D&S.

⚠ **WARNING:** *In most municipalities, the pain inflicted during S&M activities needs to be temporary and cause no significant or permanent damage to remain within legal boundaries. We encourage you to establish a set of*

RESTRAINING ORDER:

BDSM (or Bondage & Discipline, Sadism & Masochism) is a popular alternative form of sexual interfacing.

BONDAGE & DISCIPLINE
1. Restraining and punishment accessories include:

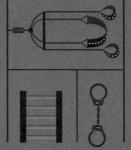

DOMINANCE & SUBMISSION
2. DOMINANT PARTNER
3. SUBMISSIVE PARTNER: Agrees to other partner's demands

SADISM & MASOCHISM
4. SADIST: inflicts pain
5. MASOCHIST: endures pain

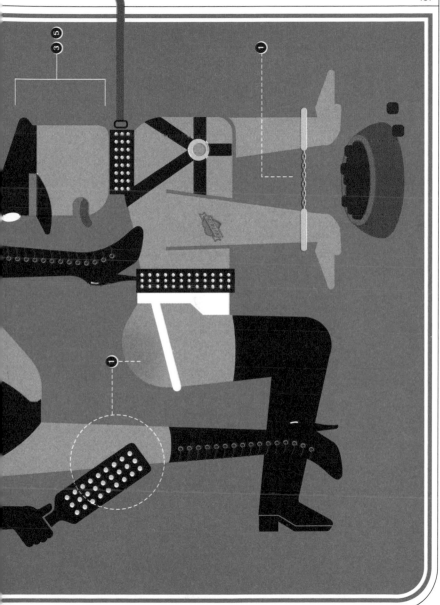

ground rules with your partner before beginning. Determine which behaviors and props are off-limits, and be sure to establish a "safe word." When engaging in S&M, cries like "no" and "stop" usually mean the exact opposite— "keep going"—so it's important to agree upon a word that's synonymous with "stop immediately." Many aficionados will use "orange" to mean "slow down" and "red" to mean "stop immediately."

Pegging: Engaging in anal intercourse with the help of a strap-on dildo (also known as performing a "strapadictomy"). The woman wears the dildo and "pegs" her male partner, who is often referred to as a "BOB," or "bend over boyfriend."

Fantasy and Role Playing: Acting out scenarios that involve sex or lead to sex in which at least one participant assumes an identity other than his or her own. Common sexual role-play scenarios include policewoman and suspect, patient and nurse/doctor, boss and secretary, repairperson and homeowner, rock star and groupie, college professor and student, and lifeguard and swimmer.

Unique Alternatives

Robotica: Engaging in sexual activity with a mechanical device not designed for sexual stimulation or a partner dressed as a cyborg.

⚠️ **WARNING:** *Be advised that most mechanical devices not designed for sexual stimulation should probably not be used for sexual stimulation. These include glass bottles, vacuum cleaners, frozen foods, and virtually anything purchased at a hardware store. Use common sense and spare yourself an embarrassing trip to the emergency room.*

Plushophilia and Furry: Deriving sexual pleasure from stuffed animals or engaging in sexual activities with someone dressed up as a giant stuffed animal.

Transophilia: Engaging in sexual activities with someone dressed as, or surgically changed into, the opposite sex that he or she was born into, or making the change yourself.

Nyctophilia: Seeking out or creating an almost completely dark environment in which to practice sexual activities.

Salirophilia: Deriving sexual pleasure from messing up your partner's hair, tearing her clothing, or covering him in mud. (Note: Careful planning for a salirophiliac encounter can help prevent the destruction of expensive bedding, clothing, and fresh perms.)

Nyotaimori: Eating sushi from the body of a naked woman. This is an ancient Japanese practice that can be adapted to participants' particular sexual and gastronomic tastes.

Macrophilia: Gaining sexual arousal from being dominated by giants, particularly Amazonian women. Can be explored through roleplay by employing costumes that include towering high heels, stilts, step ladders and tall helmets.

Determining What Turns You On

One shouldn't feel obligated to attempt any of the activities described above. If you suspect that you won't enjoy intercourse with a partner dressed as a cyborg, your instincts are probably correct. But you shouldn't feel guilty if you do enjoy these activities, and you shouldn't

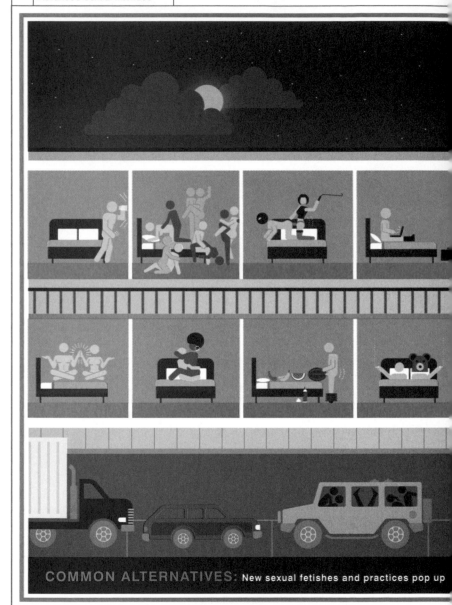

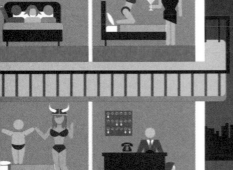

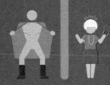

NO-TELL MOTEL

no vacancies

every day. Shown above are just a few of the possibilities.

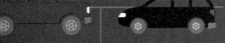

laugh at your partner if he or she proposes them. If it is legal and makes a person feel good, why not?

Also, don't be quick to dismiss all these activities as ridiculous. It's a normal reaction to laugh at any behavior that's strange or unfamiliar, but don't be surprised if one or two of these activities become lodged in your self-conscious and you find yourself dwelling upon them at random points throughout your day.

If that happens, use the Internet to gain a deeper understanding of these activities. Read stories and blog posts from other people who share your interests. Do an image search on Google (turn off the filters first). If you like what you see, try masturbating while fantasizing about performing the act yourself. Or engage in a solo simulation of the mode, as best as you can manage without hurting yourself. If, after all this, you still find yourself interested in having your partner dress as a cyborg or being covered in mud, then it's time to share your newfound interests with your partner.

Getting Your Partner on Board

Sharing your kinks with a partner can be awkward. Just because you want to make love to a giant stuffed panda bear doesn't mean your partner will be willing to invest in a giant plush panda bear costume (they're expensive, for starters, and not particularly comfortable).

But if you're in a healthy relationship, your partner will want you to be happy and sexually fulfilled. Plus, your willingness to broach the subject may encourage your partner to share his or her own strange kinks. Honest communication could lead to an improved sex life for both of you.

Use the following tips to get the ball rolling.

Reaffirm Your Attraction. Make a point to tell your partner how much you enjoy having sex together. Make him or her feel sexy and special; he or she needs to understand that you're not bored with your sex life. You're simply trying to broaden it—an admirable lifelong goal for any couple.

Watch It. Rent a Hollywood movie that incorporates some aspect of the activity into its plotline. Gauge your partner's reaction to the scenes involving the alternative. Note alternative activities in other films, books, or photographs that your partner seems to enjoy.

IF YOU'RE INTERESTED IN . . .	RENT . . .
Threesomes	*Wild Things* (1998)
Food Play	*9½ Weeks* (1986)
Voyeurism	*Rear Window* (1954)
Fashion Play	*Batman Returns* (1992)
Talking Dirty	*In the Cut* (2003)
S&M	*Secretary* (2002)

Semi-Simulate. Introduce subtle, limited versions of the activity into your regular sex play. For instance, if you are interested in B&D, try grasping your partner's wrists and gently holding down the arms during foreplay or intercourse. Gauge the reaction and gradually build on the activity in subsequent sessions.

Play Truth or Dare. Making a game of it can help introduce kink in a fun, nonthreatening way. Play your favorite card, board, video, or sports game—but make a rule that the loser will have to reveal something about his or her sexual desires. Or play a variation of strip poker, in which the loser of each hand must remove a piece of clothing. If you are honest and revealing, your partner will be emboldened to do the same.

Fantasize. Introduce the subject during a traditional session of intercourse. Ask your partner to relate a sexual fantasy while you practice his or her favorite form of stimulation. Stop and tease, saying you won't continue unless your partner reveals something new. Offer to do the same in return and subtly work the alternative activity that interests you into the narrative.

Talk About It. As a couple, have a relaxed, frank discussion about your sexual practices. Ask if he or she would like to try anything new. Let your partner know you are open to alternative desires, then ask if you can express your own. Arrange to test out both of your ideas, the sooner the better.

If your partner resists any of the techniques on this list, drop the subject and wait a few days, then broach it again using a different technique. If attempts repeatedly fail, you will need to have an open and honest conversation about your needs and desires.

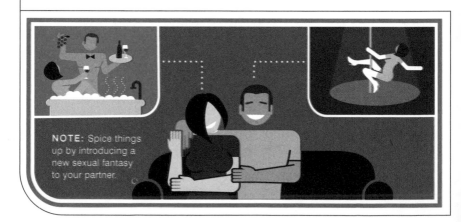

NOTE: Spice things up by introducing a new sexual fantasy to your partner.

How to Find a Third Party for a Ménage à Trois

Before you invite a third party into your bedroom, it's important to reach some conclusion with your partner about the nature and boundaries of this relationship. Your wife may be willing to share you, but only if you promise not to kiss the third party on the mouth. Your husband may be willing to share you, but only if the third party promises not to kiss him on the mouth.

Be clear, be honest, and be sure to address the following questions: Which activities are fair game? Which are off-limits? Is this a one-time experience? What will you use for contraception? Will you require the person to leave at the end of the night? It's important to listen to your spouse and respect his or her desires. Once you establish the ground rules, you can focus on selecting the ideal partner.

[1] Discuss the gender, race, and physical and personal characteristics of the third party. Some couples use their ménage à trois as an opportunity to act out long-held fantasies, such as sex with someone of a different race or socioeconomic background, or to seek out a third party who is different physically or temperamentally from their regular partner. Some men may wish to watch their partners engage in sex with someone who is better endowed, for instance, or to engage in sexual practices that are degrading or taboo. These activities may appeal to the woman as well.

[2] Make a list of potential candidates who meet all the qualifications. Begin with friends and coworkers but also consult swingers' Web sites and Internet chat rooms where like-minded folks may congregate.

TIPS FOR YOU AND YOUR PARTNER WHEN SEARCHING FOR A THIRD PERSON

1. Make a list of potential candidates and all the qualities you both are looking for in a third person.

2. The Internet is a great resource when searching for potential candidates.

3. Decide when the person will leave.

⚠ **CAUTION:** Consider eliminating candidates who are considerably more attractive than your partner.

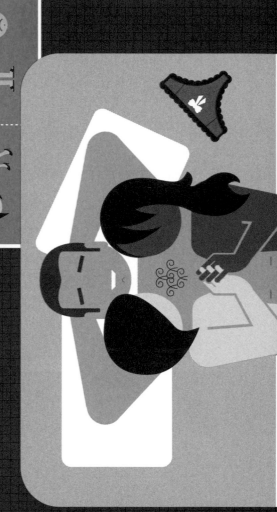

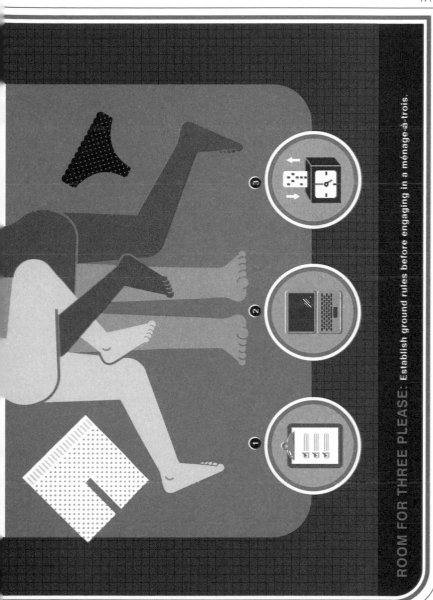

ROOM FOR THREE PLEASE: Establish ground rules before engaging in a ménage-à-trois.

[**3**] Discuss potential social and career pitfalls that could arrive from having sex with each candidate on the list. For instance, if a candidate is a coworker, determine if the encounter could negatively impact your career. Strike from the list any people who present serious pitfalls.

[**4**] Consider eliminating candidates who are considerably more attractive than your partner. Likewise, feel free to veto anyone that your partner feels strongly attracted to.

[**5**] If no names remain on the list, consider consulting personal ads to find people who match your qualifications and are also interested in engaging in a threesome.

How to Develop Your Own Alternative Sexual Activity

A week doesn't pass without some new kink or fetish popping up on the Internet—so there's no reason you can't invent your own.

[**1**] Brainstorm things or activities that you find exciting or intimidating.

[**2**] List all the aspects of that activity, including the actions and special items involved.

[**3**] Imagine how you might incorporate one aspect of the activity into sex play. For instance, if you like to play golf, imagine how you could incorporate golf equipment, such as balls, tees, and gloves, or in what places on a golf course, such as a sand trap, you could have sex.

[4] If something intimidates you, think of how you could take an aspect of it and use it as an instrument of pleasure during sex play. For instance, if you're unnerved by home repair, employ items such as a tool belt or have your partner dress as a carpenter.

[5] Try working more aspects of the person or activity into your sex play or using sexualized variations of them.

[6] If it's not turning you on, try something else.

Troubleshooting

Alternative sexual activities can lead to a host of unusual problems. Always use common sense and don't hesitate to contact medical personnel in an emergency. Here are some tips for treating a variety of lesser problems.

Overheating: People dressed in warm costumes or clothing (such as a latex dress or a giant plush panda suit) can easily overheat during the rigors of intercourse or other sexual activities. If your partner experiences dizziness, flushing, or profuse sweating, immediately remove the clothing or costume that is causing the overheating. If you cannot pull it off in the normal way and overheating continues, use scissors to gently cut your partner out of the item, being careful not to cause injury in the process. Open a window to circulate fresh air. Guide your partner into a cool bath or shower and encourage the consumption of cool water.

Skin Marking and Cutting: Paddling, spanking, whipping, and scratching can sometimes break and/or mark the skin. If the skin has been broken, apply an antibiotic ointment to prevent infection. To help fade marks, gently massage lotion into the affected areas and treat with cold compresses.

Nausea: Food play, bondage, and other activities can lead to the sense that you are about to vomit. Remove the item or stop the activity causing the nausea immediately. Get some fresh air. Try eating crackers. Suck on a lemon wedge or squeeze lemon into ice water and drink. Ginger ale and other sodas can also bring relief. If the nausea continues, it could mean you are suffering from a more serious problem. Seek medical help immediately.

Getting Lost: Lovers engaged in nyctophilia can become disoriented in near-total darkness. It's easy to get lost while returning from the bathroom or searching for an accessory in a closet. Use your voice to locate your partner, then move slowly toward the voice. Avoid long strides that might cause you to trip or step on something fragile. As you get close, ask your partner to extend his or her hands. Reach out and use the sense of touch to guide yourself to a safe location next to your partner.

Cramps: Bondage or other unfamiliar activities can cause muscular discomfort or cramps. If a position is causing pain, change it immediately (use your safe word if you require assistance). Massage the affected muscle and submerge it in warm water to relieve cramps.

Panic Attack: Any new sexual activities can be intimidating, and it's not uncommon for men and women to experience panic attacks. These are best described as a sudden onset of intense fear and anxiety; physical symptoms include trembling, faintness, cramping, nausea, and/or difficulty breathing. Victims may feel they are suffering a heart attack or other serious medical crisis. Immediately halt the activity. Turn on the lights and assure your partner that the activity has stopped. Encourage your partner to breathe deeply. Talk calmly and slowly. Offer a glass of water. Try massaging your partner's neck and shoulders (or cease all physical contact if he or she recoils from your touch). Seek medical advice even if the attack passes quickly so that you can learn the underlying causes and ways to prevent future panic attacks.

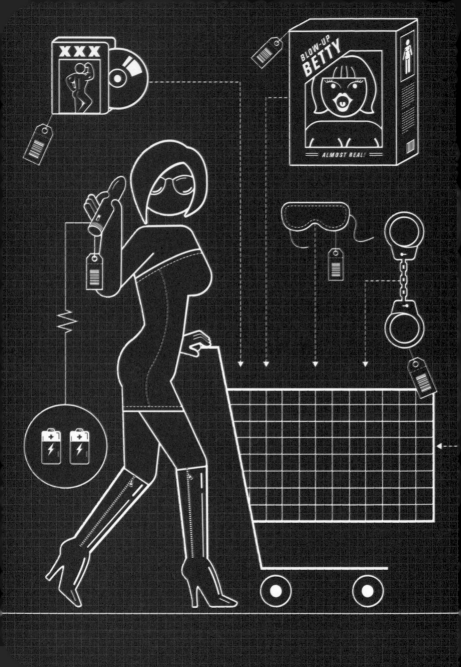

Chapter 6

Sexual
Accessories

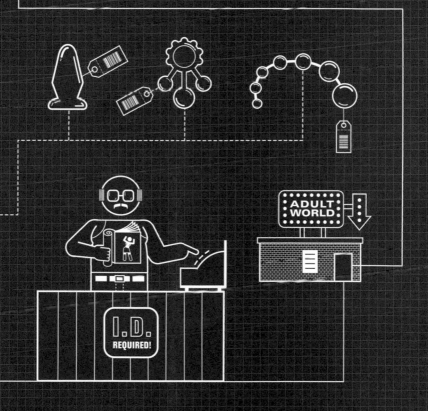

Sexual intercourse can be greatly enhanced by sexual aids, toys, and other devices. They can provide stimulation to erogenous zones that are otherwise difficult to master and may free you up to simultaneously stimulate other erogenous zones.

Be careful about introducing sexual accessories too early in a relationship. Few will prove as effective as your hands, tongue, and genitals. Plastic and rubber props can enhance any sexual experience, but they cannot substitute for a solid grounding in basic lovemaking techniques or a comprehensive knowledge of your partner's body and personal preferences.

How to Choose a Vibrator

The most popular sex toy, a vibrator quivers at varying speeds and intensities to provide stimulation to the genitals and other erogenous zones. Vibrators come in a wide variety of shapes and sizes, with some as small as a pinky and others as long and wide as a forearm; many are contoured for additional internal stimulation. Some even rotate as they quiver to add yet another stimulating motion. And since many people like to use vibrators in a bath or shower, it's easy to find one that's waterproof. Follow these steps when shopping for a vibrator—and keep in mind that you might want to own more than one.

[1] Determine what you'd like to stimulate. Vibrators intended for external use tend to have simple designs, whereas internal vibrators are shaped for easy insertion into orifices and to stimulate hard-to-reach places, such as G-spots and prostate glands within those orifices. Some are designed to simultaneously stimulate both an internal and an external erogenous zone. Other vibrators are designed for nipple stimulation, and more vigorous models can double as muscle massagers.

179

VIBRATOR WANTED: A few tips to consider before your vibrator purchase.

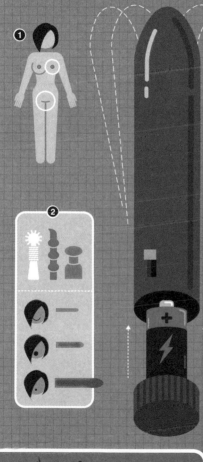

1. Consider the desired stimulation area where the vibrator will work.
2. Vibrators come in a wide variety of shapes, materials, and sizes.
3. Test a potential vibrator in an adult store or, for a more private purchase, read reviews online before you buy.
4. Always consider features that suit both you and your partner.
5. Many vibrators come disguised in other forms for privacy.

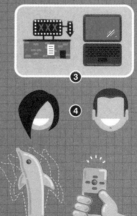

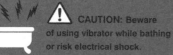

CAUTION: Beware of using vibrator while bathing or risk electrical shock.

[2] Consider your privacy needs. If you live alone, this shouldn't be an issue. But if you live with roommates, parents, or children, you may be relieved to learn that many vibrators come disguised as other objects: lipstick holders, rubber ducks, and the like.

[3] Decide if you want to use your vibrator while bathing. Many vibrators come in battery-operated, waterproof versions that are safe to use underwater. Be sure to purchase the vibrator from a reputable dealer.

[4] Pick a shape. Many vibrators are shaped like a penis, but they also come in a variety of other forms, from simple and elegant to gargantuan and silly.

[5] Decide if you want to use the vibrator solo or with a partner. If the latter, take your partner's needs and preferences into consideration. Or simply shop for a vibrator together.

[6] Rate your favorite material. Vibrators are typically made from plastic, silicone, latex, polyurethane, rubber, metal, or a jellylike substance known as polyvinyl chloride. Investigate these materials to find out which is most comfortable and to ensure that you are not allergic.

[7] Examine the vibrator before you purchase it. You'll have a difficult time finding a vibrator merchant who encourages you to try before you buy, but most respectable retailers will allow you to hold and examine different varieties. Try turning it on to get a better understanding of its intensity and how it will feel against your erogenous zones. If you don't have a nearby sex shop or boutique you feel comfortable shopping in, browse the Internet. Many sites offer detailed descriptions and even reviews of models.

[8] Compensate. If you buy a vibrator but find it unsatisfactory, you can use other materials to adjust its feel. If a vibrator proves too intense, try using it while still wearing your undergarments or a towel. A vibrator that remains too intense even through cloth can function as a muscle massager. If you don't like the material the vibrator is made from, wrap it in a condom or a swatch of soft material like silk or satin. If all else fails, buy another vibrator.

⚠ **WARNING:** *Never share sex toys with anyone except your sex partner, since they can transmit STDs. Also, be sure to clean and put them away as soon as possible after use.*

Other Sexual Accessories

There are countless other sex accessories on the market—and if you're uncomfortable walking into a retail outlet, it's now easier than ever to find these products online. Be advised that the manufacture of sex toys is not especially well regulated. This lack of oversight allows many poorly constructed items to get onto the market, some of which can be dangerous or even toxic. Try to buy your sex toys from respected manufacturers and always check to see what materials they are made from before purchasing.

Dildos and Dongs: A dildo or dong is a phallus-shaped sex toy that does not vibrate. The penislike design makes them ideal for insertion into the vagina or anus. They come in a variety of lengths, widths, contours, materials, and colors. Some dildos are double sided and designed for simultaneous insertion into two partners.

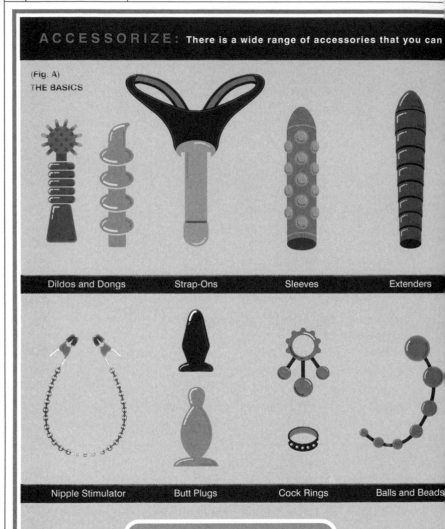

ACCESSORIZE: There is a wide range of accessories that you can

(Fig. A)
THE BASICS

Dildos and Dongs   Strap-Ons   Sleeves   Extenders

Nipple Stimulator   Butt Plugs   Cock Rings   Balls and Beads

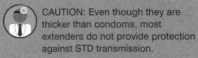

CAUTION: Even though they are thicker than condoms, most extenders do not provide protection against STD transmission.

mploy to heighten the sexual interface experience for you and your partner.

ig. B)
AFETY AND COMFORT:

1 Condoms
2 Lubricants

AFTER DARK CONDOMS
NEW!
GLOWS IN THE DARK!
(1)

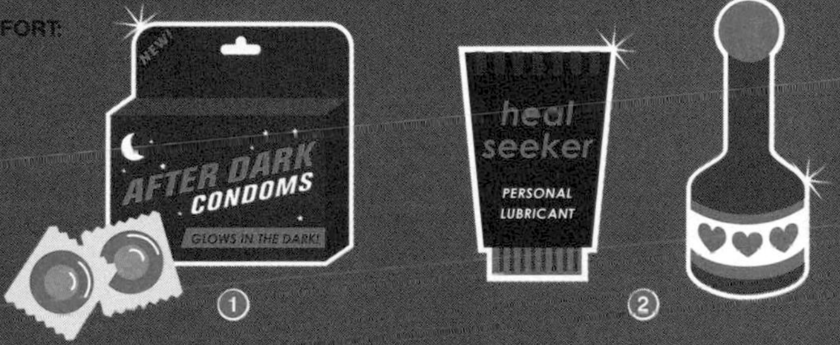

heal seeker
PERSONAL LUBRICANT
(2)

Fig. C)
RESTRAIN YOURSELF

1 Swings
2 Restraints
3 Blindfolds

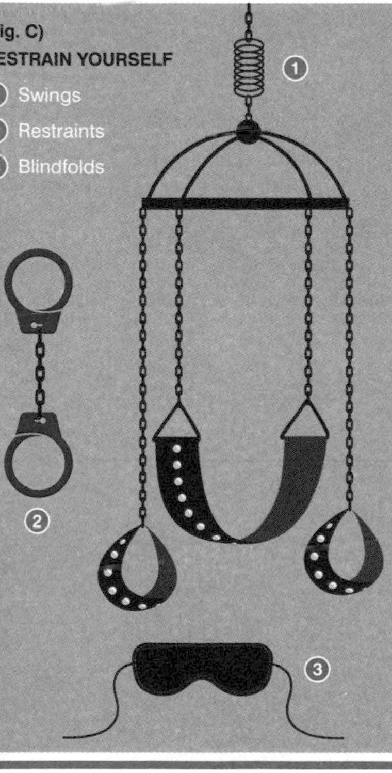

(Fig. D)
HOUSEHOLD ITEMS THAT CAN BE USED
AS SEXUAL-ACCESSORY SUBSTITUTES

1 Shower Nozzle
2 Cell Phone (in vibrate mode)
3 Pillows
4 Gloves

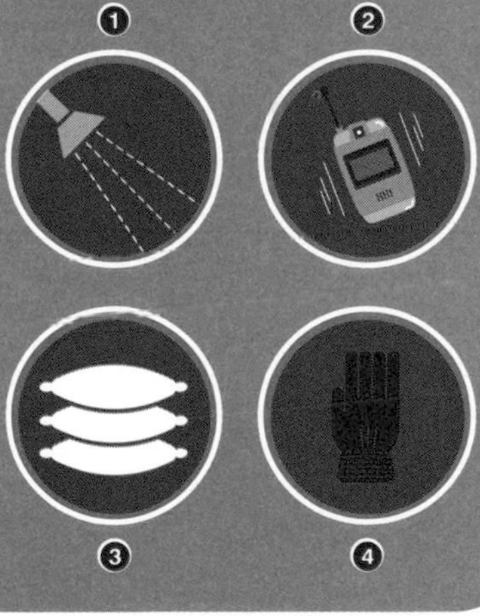

Strap-Ons: These dildos come attached to a belt so that you can thrust with them as you would a real penis. They make a good aid for men with erection problems or for anyone looking to experience penetration from the other side.

Sleeves: Just as the dildo serves as a surrogate penis, the sleeve acts as a substitute orifice to insert the penis into and simulate the act of intercourse.

Extenders: These dildolike items have a hollow interior, allowing men wanting to add a few inches to slip their penises inside and then engage in intercourse.

⚠ *WARNING: Though they tend to be five to ten times thicker than a condom, most extenders do not provide an effective barrier against STD transmission. Wear a condom over them. Doing so will also help keep the extender from falling off during thrusting.*

Nipple Stimulators: Clamps and rings designed for attachment to the nipples offer intense stimulation for these highly charged erogenous zones.

Butt Plugs: These short, relatively thin, phallus-shaped items are designed to be inserted into the anus and kept there for several minutes or even hours. Some come with vibrating capabilities for added stimulation.

Condoms and Lubes: These can not only help protect you from sexually transmitted disease, discomfort, and injury, they enhance pleasure as well. (For a full discussion of condoms and specialty condoms, see pages 109–118.)

Cock Rings: These doughnut-shaped items slip over the top of a penis and slide down to its base to help trap blood in the shaft and glans, helping to create and sustain an erection while enhancing sensitivity.

Balls and Beads: Attached to a string, these items are inserted into the vagina or anus for exercises to tighten muscles, solo stimulation, or extra sensation during intercourse.

Swings: Harnessed to a door or beam, these support systems allow one partner to sit comfortably and securely during intercourse, creating possibilities for new angles and positions.

⚠️ **WARNING:** *Do not attempt to use a child's swing set for sexual play. The toy swing may break due to overstrain from supporting an adult body and result in injury to the back, genitals, and other hardware.*

Restraints: Modeled after handcuffs, these gadgets loop around the wrists or ankles during bondage sex play.

Blindfolds: A common item in bondage play, blindfolds can also be employed by couples looking to heighten the sensation of touch during interface by temporarily blocking the sense of sight.

Everyday Items That Can Be Used as Sexual Accessories

- Shower Nozzle (to squirt water onto erogenous zones)
- Cell Phone (as vibrator substitute)
- Feather Duster (for stimulation)
- Pillow (to change angles during intercourse)
- Hammock (for new intercourse positions)
- Ice Cubes (to change temperature and heighten sensation during foreplay)
- Gloves (to alter sensation of touch)
- Bandana (as blindfold or restraint)

Caring for Your Accessories

Well-manufactured sex accessories come with information about the materials they are made from and detailed maintenance instructions. Even those that don't come with clear directions need to be maintained as well as possible. Some toys are made of materials that can break down when subjected to lubricants. Others can develop nicks or cracks that could lead to painful injuries. Maintain your sex toys in good condition—for the sake of the toy as well as your own health.

[1] Follow the maintenance instructions. If the accessory came without such instructions, find out what material it is made from and research the best way to maintain it. Plastic, latex, and silicone require different maintenance techniques. Learn what your toy needs to stay in tip-top shape.

[2] Make sure you use the correct lube. Some materials break down quick-ly when subjected to silicone and other substances commonly found in lubes. Read the label to see what material your sex toy is made from and read the ingredients label of your lube to ensure that they work well together.

[3] Clean after use. Sex toys will be subjected to potentially damaging flu-ids and other substances during sex. They may even pick up an STD from your partner. Clean them thoroughly with hot, soapy water or whatever cleaning substance is best suited for the material. Then dry thoroughly and even powder with cornstarch. Some materials break down when subjected to moisture of any kind over a long period of time.

[4] Watch out for lint. Small bits of fuzz and similar materials tend to stick to certain sex toy materials. Make sure your sex toy remains lint free.

[5] Store properly. Keep your sex toys in a dark, dry, sturdy container. Sunlight, moisture, and exposure can weaken the material many sex toys are made from. Also make sure your storage container cannot be invaded by kids, pets, or nosy roommates.

[6] If you own a vibrator or other device with a motor, periodically inspect its wires to make sure they aren't becoming frayed or loosened. If the item runs on batteries, check them for signs of corrosion and replace if necessary.

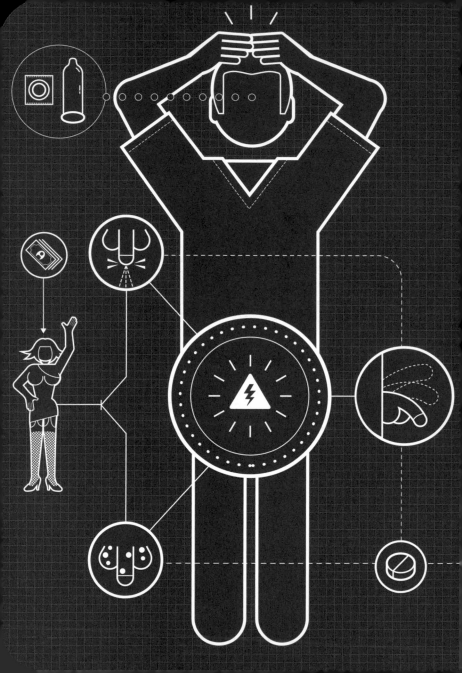

Chapter 7

Maintenance and Troubleshooting

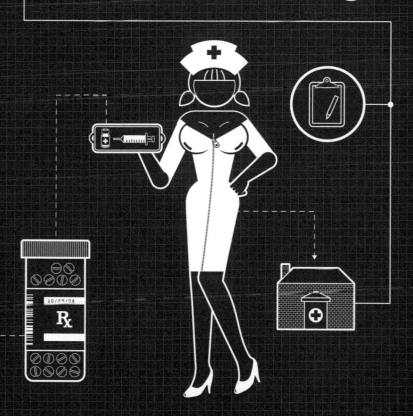

Even if you achieve a consistently satisfying level of sexual activity, it's important to take regular actions to maintain the relationship, and remain vigilant for any warning signs of trouble.

Hardware Maintenance

Keeping your hardware in good condition improves not only your chances of peak sexual performance but also the chances that your partner will continue wanting to interface with you.

A regular exercise program that combines cardio workouts and muscle building and toning exercises will provide a sound base. Feel free to add a few exercises designed specifically for hardware parts that are key to sexual attraction and interface.

Glute Lifts: Your buttocks muscles, or glutes, play a big role in intercourse and in helping you to look attractive. This simple exercise tones them and provides a workout for your abs and legs. Lie with your back on the ground and your arms on either side of your torso. Bend your knees and place your feet on the ground beneath them, about hip-width apart. Squeeze your buttocks muscles together as you lift them off the ground, leaving only your feet, shoulders, and head on the ground. Hold for three seconds and return your buttocks to the floor. Repeat 10 times.

The Plank: This pose will stretch and strengthen all the core muscles, which are key to intercourse and many other sexual activities. Lie on your stomach, with your legs extended straight behind you, supporting yourself on your forearms and elbows, which are bent under your shoulders. Curl your toes beneath you to rise up slightly and then straighten your arms as though doing a push-up, creating a flat line, or plank, from your head to your heels.

Distribute your weight evenly between your toes and forearms. Engage your abs, back, and buttocks muscles, holding yourself in this position as long as you can or up to a minute.

Love-Handle Toner: Though they have a nice-sounding name, love handles (the bulges of fat just above your hips) don't look terribly attractive or provide a comfortable handle to grab onto during lovemaking. Reducing and toning them will help make your midriff stronger, more flexible, and more attractive, but simple weight loss won't necessarily get rid of them.

Pec Builders: The chest serves as a hardware focal point for both males and females. Keeping your chest muscles, or pecs, toned will help sustain your sex appeal and aid in sexual performance. Grab dumbbells that you can comfortably hold in each hand, straddle a weight bench, and lie back with your feet flat on the floor to each side. Position the dumbbells over your nipples, with your palms facing each other. Simultaneously press them upward, rotating your wrists as you go so your palms are facing your knees as you reach the top. Concentrate on making your pecs do most of the work, not your arms, squeezing them together slightly as you lift. Return the dumbbells to the starting position by your nipples, then repeat as many times as you can. To emphasize the upper pecs, perform this exercise on a weight bench slanted at approximately a 45-degree angle.

Kegels: Named for Dr. Arthur Kegel, these exercises strengthen the PC muscles near the genitals. They can augment sexual gratification, increase vaginal and anal tightness, ease pains during pregnancy, and help men with ejaculation problems (see "Premature Ejaculation," page 196). Acquire a book, video, or other instructional item that explains how to perform kegels. Or consult with your genital hardware service provider for more information.

Additional Maintenance

Masturbation: Your genitals require regular workouts to remain fit, just like the rest of your hardware. Apply the Manual Genitalia Manipulation techniques outlined in chapter 3 on yourself. You can also use a vibrator, sleeve, or one of the other accessories discussed in chapter 6.

Wardrobe Upgrades: Most people see you and rate your sexual interface appeal only while you are fully clothed. Even your regular interface partner sees you much more often in clothes than out of them. So what you wear—and the resulting effects on the presentation of your hardware and software—plays a huge role in your sex life. Regularly add new looks and clothing that make you appealing in new ways. Try changing hairstyles and colognes or perfumes. Test out undergarments designed to enhance the appeal of your key sexual hardware.

Makeover: If you feel like you've hit a dead end in your sex appeal, try a complete and fundamental change in your wardrobe, hairstyle, makeup, and every other aspect of your visual appearance. The "new you" will likely attract new interface partners or renewed interest from an existing partner. Consult an exterior hardware designer, aka a makeover specialist, for help.

Software Maintenance and Upgrades: Your attitude and personality can bolster or undermine your physical appearance and sex appeal. Audit your interactions with potential and existing sex partners to make sure you haven't fallen into dull, predictable patterns or negative dynamics. Refresh your personality by learning new things or trying something you have always wanted to do.

ADDITIONAL MAINTENANCE REQUIRED

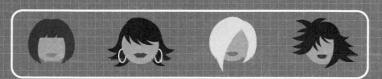

MAINTENANCE MODIFICATIONS

1. Stoke your fire by practicing masturbation.

2. Get a makeup and hair makeover to discover a "new you."

3. Try upgrading your wardrobe to feel sexier.

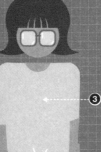

Black Beauty

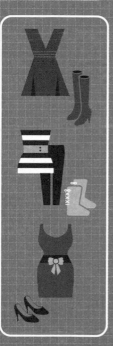

NOTE: Trying new things can refresh your personality and instill you with an inner confidence that can bolster your overall sex appeal to others.

Relationship Maintenance

Relationships invariably encounter difficulties or tedium. If you think you and your partner have fundamental problems, consult a certified software specialist, aka a marriage counselor or psychologist.

You can also try defragging your software with tactics that you can employ on your own and with the help of your partner.

Travel: Experience new places together. It will help you see each other differently or remind you of your original attraction.

Shared Hobby: Take up a new recreational activity together. It will reinvigorate your attraction while developing new skills and interests together.

Perspective: It can be difficult for partners to recall their initial attraction after a prolonged period of intimate interaction. Watch others interact with your partner during social or work gatherings. Note the aspects of your partner that appeal to others—qualities you may have overlooked or forgotten.

Talk: Explore new conversation topics to get to know aspects of your partner's software programming. Find playful ways to share unexplored aspects of your lives, desires, and fears.

Snuggle: Spend more time in bed or on a couch hugging and holding and just being next to each other. This activity can build trust, intimacy, and attraction.

Massage: Take a course, get a book, or watch a video about sensual massage. Then practice it on each other. Massage relaxes and resets the muscles, often working out software bugs that are hindering your mutual interactions. It is also highly pleasurable.

Foreplay: Spend more time in foreplay mode, especially the initial touching stage. Dedicate entire sexual interface sessions to foreplay or just initial touching without moving on to genital manipulation. It will help you build appreciation and understanding of the other's hardware and software programming.

Afterplay: Take time after your sexual interface sessions to snuggle, talk, perform initial touching exercises, and generally increase trust and intimacy.

Mutual Masturbation: Watching each other masturbate can teach you new techniques for pleasuring your partner. Discussing erotically activating topics during these exercises can also help expand your understanding of your partner's erotic software.

Experiment: Expand your interface horizons by trying some of the intercourse positions (see chapter 4). Or try an alternative method of sexual interface (see chapter 5).

Addressing Sexual Malfunctions

Many persons suffer hardware and software malfunctions that directly disrupt sexual interface. You can attempt to overcome and cure the problems, but many require consultation with a service provider.

Erectile Dysfunction: The inability to achieve genital activation (also known as impotence or a "lack of lead in the pencil") ranks as one of the most common and debilitating male sexual malfunctions. It happens occasionally to almost every man; those who experience it may feel shame and fail to take steps to address the problem. If you or your partner encounters repeated episodes of erectile dysfunction, it could indicate circulation problems, diabetes, or another serious medical situation. Consult with a physician as soon as possible.

General Sexual Dysfunction (GSD): Formally known as "frigidity," GSD affects persons who cannot orgasm and/or feel significant desire for or enjoyment from sex. The causes and cures of this condition can be quite simple or complex and involve any number of physical and psychological issues. Seek professional help as soon as possible and consider couples counseling.

Premature Ejaculation: The most common male genital malfunction causes the male to ejaculate in the early stages of sexual interface, before he or his partner can gain full satisfaction. While premature ejaculation happens occasionally to almost every male, those who experience it often feel shame and fail to take steps to address the problem. If you or your partner encounters repeated episodes of premature ejaculation, try these methods.

■ *Masturbation Practice:* Most men can condition themselves away from premature ejaculation through practice during masturbation. Just stimulate yourself slowly, pausing just before orgasm. Wait until the urge to orgasm passes, then repeat as many times as you can handle. Repeat this exercise several times a week. By delaying orgasm, you will help condition your penis and brain to handle more prolonged periods of stimulation before orgasm.

■ *Desensitizing Lubricants:* Some specialty lubricants limit the stimulation of the penis during intercourse, helping males delay orgasm.

■ *Condoms:* Many condoms, particularly thicker varieties, limit stimulation of the penis during intercourse, helping males delay orgasm.

■ *Kegels:* These exercises strengthen the PC muscles by your genitals that can help curtail ejaculation. Acquire a book, video, or other instructional item that explains how to perform kegels. Or you can consult with your genital hardware service provider for more information.

■ *Mind over Matter:* You may find that thinking about sporting events, unattractive celebrities, or mundane day-to-day tasks serves as an effective curb to premature ejaculation. However, an unfortunate by-product of this technique may be the loss of erection entirely.

If you continue to experience repeated episodes of premature ejaculation, consult with a physician, psychological professional, or faith leader.

TIME YOUR STAMINA:

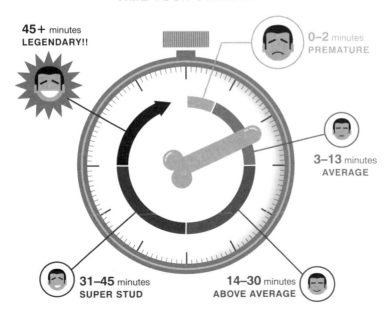

Malware: Sexually Transmitted Diseases

Dozens of different infections can be passed between partners during sexual interface. Some lead to inconvenience and embarrassment, but others can disfigure and even kill. Using condoms can prevent the spread of STDs, but it is not a guarantee.

Your best defense against STDs remains information and caution. So although it may not seem to be a particularly seductive activity, you need to hold a frank and thorough discussion with potential partners before engaging in even the early phases of interface. Ask if they have any STDs, the last time they were tested, and if they have had any new interface partners since their last testing. Let them know it is a deadly serious matter and you are holding them accountable for being honest and forthright.

STDs sometimes manifest themselves with sores, blisters, swelling, discharges, rashes, warts, and insectlike creatures in pubic hair. If you spot any of these on your partner, immediately postpone sexual interface activity and demand that he or she get a full medical checkup.

If you have any of these symptoms yourself, or experience unexplained abdominal pain, discomfort during urination, or discolored or foul-smelling discharge, seek immediate medical attention.

You should also get regularly tested for common STDs such as HIV/AIDS, herpes, and genital warts. Some STDs can be treated quickly, whereas others stay with you for life. The best treatment is not to contract them in the first place.

FOR OFFICE USE ONLY

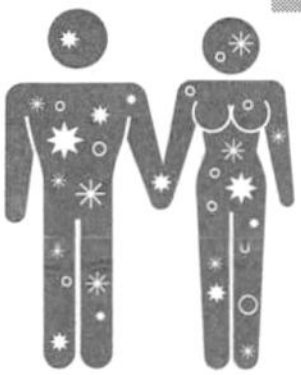

USE THIS HANDY CHECKLIST TO SPOT SIGNS OF AN STD IN YOUR PARTNER.

NOTE: Condoms can help prevent the spread of STDs

	IF YOU SEE . . .	THEN HE/SHE MAY HAVE . . .	TREATABLE:	CURABLE:
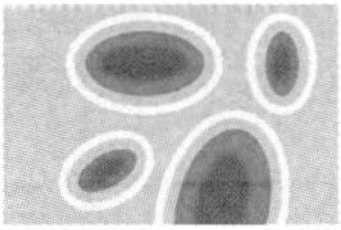	Oval, buttonlike sores on the genitals or rectum	**Syphilis**	Y	Y
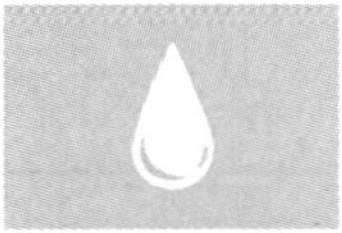	Puslike penile discharge	**Gonorrhea**	Y	Y
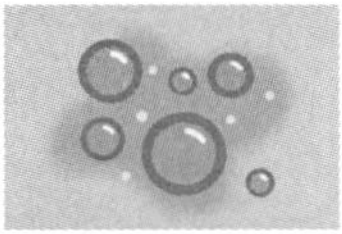	Crusty genital blisters	**Herpes**	Y	N
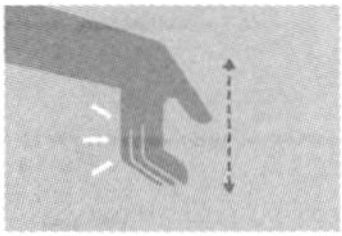	Persistent scratching of genital area	**Pubic Lice** (aka crabs)	Y	Y
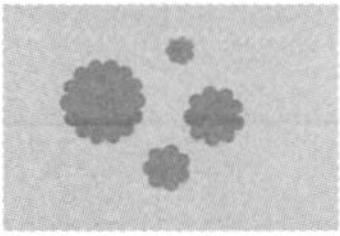	Small, flesh-colored lumps with cauliflower appearance	**Human Papillomavirus**	Y	N

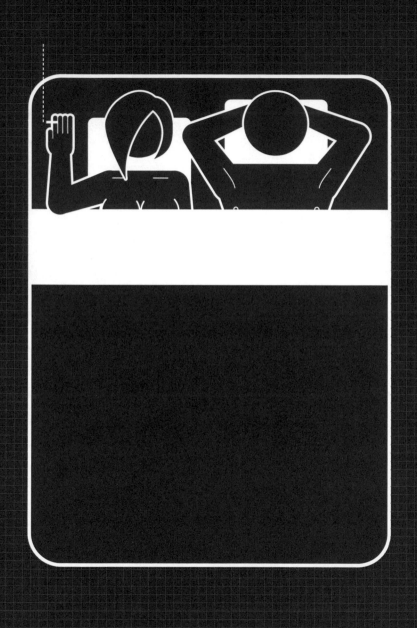

[Appendix]

Technical Support

The following organizations offer a variety of information and services.

Centers for Disease Control and Prevention
(800) 232-4636
http://www.cdc.gov/STD/
U.S. government agency dedicated to the study and control of disease, including STDs, and to educating the public.

The Kinsey Institute
(812) 855-7686
http://www.indiana.edu/~kinsey/
Academic center for multifaceted research on human sexuality.

Planned Parenthood
1-800-230-PLAN
http://www.plannedparenthood.org/
Provides information on sexuality, health, and reproductivity issues for women.

The Sinclair Institute
(800) 855-0888
http://www.sinclairinstitute.com/
A source of scholarly research and advice on sexual matters as well as instructional videos and books and other sexual aides.

Dan Savage
http://www.thestranger.com/seattle/savagelove
National syndicated sex columnist who offers advice on a wide range of sex topics in print, online, in lectures, and through regular podcasts.

Index

Page numbers in *italics* indicate illustrations.

A

accessories, sexual, 178–87, *182–83*
Adams apple, 45
air embolism, 93
anal intercourse, 141–44, *143*, 162
aphrodisiacs, 22–23
arms, 15, 39

B

back, 39
balls and beads, 185
B&D (bondage and discipline), 159
BDSM (bondage, discipline, sadism, and masochism), 159, *160–61*
beds, 100–102. *See also* waterbeds
birth control pills, 120
blindfolds, 185
body parts, 10–15, *12–13*. *See also specific parts*
body preparation, 25–33
bondage and discipline (B&D), 159
booting up, 36–40
brassieres, 46
breasts, 14, 46–50, *47*
butt plugs, 184
buttocks, 44

C

cervical caps, 119
cervical sponges, 119
cervix, 66
circumcision, 57
climax, male, 78, *78*. *See also* ejaculation; orgasms
clitoral hood, 63, 96
clitoris, 65, 84–85, 96
clothing and accessories, 29–33, *30–31*, 192
cock rings, 185
coconuts, 22
co-eating, 51
condoms, 109–19, *114–15*, *118*, 184, 196, 198
coronal ridge, 60
cuddling, 38
cunnilingus, 92–97
cutting, 173–74
cybersex, 154–55

D

dental dams, 97
diaphragms, 119–20
dildos, 181
dirty talk, 158
dominance and submission (D&S), 159
dongs, 181
D&S (dominance and submission), 159
durian, 22–23

E

ears, 14
edible underwear, 51
ejaculation, 78–79, 149, 196, *197*
erectile dysfunction, 195–96
exercises, 25–27, 190–91
exhibitionism, 159
extenders (penis), 61, 184
eyes, 14

F

fantasies, 162, 168
fashion play, 155, *156–57*
feet, 15, 26, 40, 155
fellatio, 86–92
fetishes, 155
fingers, 15
food and food play, 22–23, 158, 163
foreplay, 41–44, 46–51, *52–53*, 195
foreskin, 57
frenulum, 60

G

general sexual dysfunction (GSD), 196
genitalia. *See also specific parts*
    female, 63–67, *64*, 79–85, 92–97
    male, 56–62, *58–59*, 71–79,
      72–73, 86–92, *88–89*
    malfunctions of, 61–62
    manipulation, female, 79–85
    manipulation, male, 71–79
glans, 57
Gräfenberg, Ernst, 66
groin, 25
group sex, 155, 169–72

GSD (general sexual dysfunction), 196
G-spot, 66, 96

H

hair, 10, 40, 48. *See also* pubic hair
hands, 15, 39
head, 10
hickies, 45
home preparation, 18–19, *20–21*
hygiene, 28, *30–31*, 52–53, 85
hymen, 66
hypospadias, 62

I

impotence, 195–96
initialization (seduction), 36–40
intercourse, anal, 141–44, *143*, 162
intercourse, sexual. *See also* sexual
    interface, advanced
      accessories and, 178–87, *182–83*
      anal intercourse, 141–44, *143*, 162
      essential items, 102–7
      mechanics, 121
      menstruation and, 140
      positions, 124–39
      protective devices, 109–20
      songs, appropriate, 106
      work stations, 100, *104–5*

K

Kegel, Arthur, 191
kegels, 191, 196–97
kissing, 41–44, *42*
knees, 44

L

labia majora, 63
labia minora, 63
legs, 15, 26
lips, 43–44
lubrication, 48, 68–71, *70*, 184, 196

M

macrophilia, 163
malfunctions, genital, 61–62
malfunctions, sexual, 195–97
massages, 37–38, 150, 194
masturbation, 192, 195, 196
ménage à trois, 155, 169–72, *170–71*
menstruation, 140
micropenis, 61
midriff, 44
mons, 65
mouth, 27. *See also* kissing

N

neck, 14, 25, 45
nipple stimulators, 184
nose, 14
nyctophilia, 163, 174
nyotaimori, 163

O

oral interface, 41–44, *42*
oral-genital interface
      female genitalia and, 92–97, *94–95*
      hygiene and, 85
      male genitalia and, 86–92, *88–89*
orgasms, 144–51, *146. See also*
   climax, male; ejaculation

orgies, 155
oysters, 22

P

panic attacks, 174–75
pegging, 162
penile enhancement, 60–61
penis. See genitalia
penis, strap-on-synthetic, 141
penis curvature, 61
perineum, 76
Peyronie's diesease, 61
phimosis, 62
physical appearance, *24*, 192
plushophilia, 163
premature ejaculation, 196, *197*
priapism, 62
prophylactics, 109–20, *114–15*, *117*,
   184, 196, 198
prostate, 142
P-Spot, 142
pubic hair, 60, 65, 67

R

relationships, maintenance of, 194–95
remote sex, 154
restraints, 185
robotica, 162
role playing, 162
rubbers, 109–19

S

sadism and masochism (S&M), 159, 162
salirophilia, 163
scrotum, 60

seduction, 22–23, 36–40

seduction aids, consumable, 22–23

semen, 90–91

sex, remote, 154

sexual accessories, 178–87, *182-183*

sexual intercourse. *See* intercourse, sexual

sexual interface, advanced

    alternatives, 154–63, *164–65*

    books depicting, 158

    developing your own, 172–73

    films depicting, 158, 167

    partners and, 166–68

    preferences, 163, 166

    troubleshooting, 173–75

sexual malfunctions, 195–97

sexually transmitted diseases (STDs), 198–99

shaft, 57, 60

shoes, 32

shoulders, 14, 39

skin, 14, 32

skin marking, 173

sleeves, 184

S&M (sadism and masochism), 159, 162

Spanish fly, 23

sperm, 91

spermicide, 119

STDs (sexually transmitted diseases), 198–99

stomach, 15

strapadictomy, 141, 162, 184

strap-on-synthetic penis, 141, 162, 184

swings, 185

T

talking dirty, 158

tantric sex, 158

thighs, 45

threesomes. *See* ménage à trois

tongue, 27, 43

touching, 39–40, 44–45

transophilia, 163

truffles, 22

U

underwear, 29, 51

urethra, female, 65

urethra, male, 57

V

vagina, 66

vasectomies, 120

vibrators, 150, 178–81, *179*

visual cues, 38

vocalization, 151

voyeurism, 159

W

wakame sake, 158

warm-ups, 25–27

waterbeds, 102

Y

yeast infections, 51, 68, 111

SEXUAL CERTIFICATE

Congratulations! Now that you've studied all the instructions in this manual, you are fully prepared to engage in a pleasurable and active sex life. With a little creativity, dedication, and practice, you can enjoy a lifetime of sexual bliss.

Your Name

Your Partner's Name

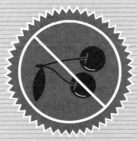

Your Favorite Position

Your Partner's Favorite Position

Your Sexual Fantasy

Your Partner's Sexual Fantasy

About the Author

FELICIA ZOPOL is the author of several books including *The 10 Secrets to Great Sex* and *Let's Talk about Sex: More Than 600 Quotes on the World's Oldest Obsession*. She served as the sex and relationships columnist for Dreamlife, Inc.

About the Illustrators

PAUL KEPPLE and **SCOTTY REIFSNYDER** are better known as the Philadelphia-based studio **HEADCASE DESIGN**. Their work has been featured in many design and illustration publications, such as *AIGA 365* and *50 Books/50 Covers, American Illustration*, *Communication Arts*, and *Print*. Paul worked at Running Press Book Publishers for several years before opening Headcase in 1998. He graduated from the Tyler School of Art, where he now teaches. Scotty is a graduate of Kutztown University and received his M.F.A. from Tyler School of Art, where he had Paul as an instructor.